Physical Therapy for Traumatic Brain Injury

CLINICS IN PHYSICAL THERAPY

EDITORIAL BOARD

Physical Therapy for the Cancer Patient
Charles L. McGarvey III, M.S., P.T., guest editor

Gait in Rehabilitation
Gary L. Smidt, Ph.D., guest editor

Physical Therapy of the Hip
John L. Echternach, Ed.D., guest editor

Physical Therapy of the Shoulder, 2nd Ed.
Robert Donatelli, M.A., P.T., guest editor

Pediatric Neurologic Physical Therapy, 2nd Ed.
Suzann K. Campbell, Ph.D., P.T., F.A.P.T.A., guest editor

Physical Therapy Management of Parkinson's Disease
George I. Turnbull, M.A., P.T., guest editor

Pulmonary Management in Physical Therapy
Cynthia Coffin Zadai, M.S., P.T., guest editor

Physical Therapy Assessment in Early Infancy
Irma J. Wilhelm, M.S., P.T., guest editor

Physical Therapy of the Low Back, 2nd Ed.
Lance T. Twomey, Ph.D., and James R. Taylor, M.D.,
Ph.D., guest editors

Temporomandibular Disorders, 2nd Ed.
Steven L. Kraus, P.T., guest editor

Physical Therapy of the Cervical and Thoracic Spine, 2nd Ed.
Ruth Grant, B.P.T., M.App.Sc., Grad.Dip.Adv.Man.Ther., guest editor

Forthcoming Volumes in the Series

Physical Therapy of the Knee, 2nd Ed.
Robert E. Mangine, M.Ed., P.T., A.T.C., guest editor

Physical Therapy of the Foot and Ankle, 2nd Ed.
Gary C. Hunt, M.A., P.T., O.C.S., and
Thomas G. McPoil, Ph.D., P.T., A.T.C., guest editors

Physical Therapy for Traumatic Brain Injury

Edited by

Jacqueline Montgomery, P.T.

Clinical Professor
Department of Biokinesiology and Physical Therapy
University of Southern California
Los Angeles, California
Director
Department of Physical Therapy
Rancho Los Amigos Medical Center
Downey, California

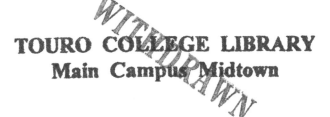

CHURCHILL LIVINGSTONE
New York, Edinburgh, London, Madrid, Melbourne, Milan, Tokyo

midtown

Library of Congress Cataloging-in-Publication Data

Physical therapy for traumatic brain injury / edited by Jacqueline
  Montgomery.
        p.   cm. — (Clinics in physical therapy)
     Includes bibliographical references and index.
     ISBN 0-443-08908-6
     1.   Brain damage—Physical therapy. I. Montgomery, Jacqueline.
  II. Series.
   [DNLM: 1. Brain Injuries—rehabilitation. 2. Physical Therapy.
  WL 354 P578 1995]
  RC387.5.P48   1995
  617.4′8106—dc20
  DNLM/DLC
  for Library of Congress   94-30223
                                                                 CIP

Distributed in the United Kingdom by Churchill Livingstone, Robert Stevenson House, 1–3
Baxter's Place, Leith Walk, Edinburgh EH1 3AF, and by associated companies, branches, and
representatives throughout the world.

The Publishers have made every effort to trace the copyright holders for borrowed material. If
they have inadvertently overlooked any, they will be pleased to make the necessary
arrangements at the first opportunity.

Acquisitions Editor: *Carol Bader*
Copy Editor: *Elizabeth Bowman-Schulman*
Production Supervisor: *Patricia McFadden*

Printed in the United States of America

First published in 1995   7 6 5 4 3 2 1

In loving memory of
my mother and father
who encouraged me at every turn,
modeled for me the values of learning,
insisted on always striving for excellence,
and instilled the constant strength
and beauty of the written word.

*"Always maintain your passion
for your life's work."*

Contributors

DeAnna Anderson, P.T.
Adjunct Instructor, Department of Biokinesiology and Physical Therapy, University of Southern California, Los Angeles, California; Neurologic Resource Clinician/PT II, Physical Therapy Department, Rancho Los Amigos Medical Center, Downey, California

Mei Lee Chiu, P.T.
Instructor, Department of Physical Therapy, Loma Linda University, Loma Linda, California; Physical Therapy Instructor/Senior Clinician, Department of Physical Therapy, Rancho Los Amigos Medical Center, Downey, California

Beth Fisher, M.S., P.T., N.C.S.
Doctoral Student, Department of Biokinesiology and Physical Therapy, University of Southern California, Los Angeles, California; Neurologic Clinical Specialist, Department of Physical Therapy, Rancho Los Amigos Medical Center, Downey, California

Douglas E. Garland, M.D.
Clinical Professor, Department of Orthopaedic Surgery, University of Southern California School of Medicine, Los Angeles, California; Chief, Neurotrauma Services, Department of Surgery, Rancho Los Amigos Medical Center, Downey, California

Kathleen Gill-Body, M.S., P.T., N.C.S.
Assistant Professor, Graduate Program in Physical Therapy, Massachusetts General Hospital Institute of Health Professions; Neurologic Clinical Specialist, Physical Therapy Services, Massachusetts General Hospital, Boston, Massachusetts

Marie Magliozzi Giorgetti, M.S., P.T., N.C.S.
Adjunct Instructor, Graduate Program in Physical Therapy, Massachusetts General Hospital Institute of Health Professions; Clinical Specialist, Physical Therapy Services, Massachusetts General Hospital, Boston, Massachusetts

John F. O'Leary, Ph.D.
Clinical Director, Haggerty Center for Neurorehabilitation, Northville, Michigan

Mitchell Rosenthal, Ph.D.
Vice President, Research and Education, Rehabilitation Institute of Michigan, Detroit, Michigan

Katherine Sullivan, M.S., P.T.
Teaching Assistant, Department of Biokinesiology and Physical Therapy, University of Southern California, Los Angeles, California

Cynthia Stone Thomas, P.T.
Adjunct Faculty, Physical Therapy Program in Clinical Applications of Neuroscience, Texas Woman's University Graduate School of Health Sciences, Dallas, Texas; Director, Equest Hippotherapy Program, Dallas, Texas; Physical Therapy Consultant, Centrode Aprendizaje, Cuernavaca, Mexico; Private Practice, Dallas, Texas

Jan Utley, P.T.
Adjunct Faculty, Physical Therapy Program in Clinical Applications of Neuroscience, Texas Woman's University Graduate School of Health Sciences, Dallas, Texas; Private Practice, Dallas-Fort Worth, Texas; Coordinator of continuing education workshops for clinicians in management of brain-injured adults in the United States, Canada, and Europe

Susan Woll, P.T.
Private Practice, Denver, Colorado

Cynthia M. Zablotny, M.S., P.T., N.C.S.
Clinical Instructor, Department of Physical Therapy, Ithaca College; Staff Physical Therapist, Brain Injury Rehabilitation Program, St. Mary's Hospital, Rochester, New York

Preface

Even the most seasoned clinician appreciates the complexity of treating the traumatically brain-injured adult. It can be one of the most daunting of diagnostic patient categories a therapist encounters. Aberrant behavioral and cognitive sequelae as well as significant physical manifestations result from injury to and involvement of multiple systems. The knowledge base and skills acquisition required to manage this patient population artfully and successfully is a continual challenge in career development.

In *Physical Therapy for Traumatic Brain Injury*, acknowledged experts and certified specialists, some of whom have devoted entire careers to the study of and treatment development for those with head injury, share their considerable expertise and experience. The information they share ranges from acute management to reintegration of the patient into meaningful living and lifestyles.

The content was designed to be applicable to the neophyte as well as the practicing clinician. Topics reflect contemporary, state-of-the-art, efficacious rehabilitation techniques (Chapters 1, 4, 5, and 6). In Chapters 2 and 3, the authors include current techniques and theories and also propose original applications or modified approaches to treatment (both cognitive and for improving motor control) based on their studies and experiences. Chapter 7 provides a unique and contemporary orthotic management approach for the lower limb. Chapters 8, 9, and 10 take us out of the direct realm of physical therapy. The authors, leaders and brain-injury trailblazers in their fields of medicine (surgery) and neuropsychology, respectively, provide information and management approaches for the "complete clinician" to consider and incorporate into a repertoire for the management of the patient with head injury.

Today, fewer people are being injured (and the injuries are less severe) in motor vehicle accidents. This decline, presumably, is a result of automobile seat belt laws and improved safety restraints, regulations for helmet use by bicycle and motorcycle riders, and massive public campaigns to deter alcohol use combined with driving. Unfortunately these numbers are quickly being filled by those injured from the increasing incidence of violence throughout the country. Indeed, over the nine-year period through 1992, admissions for gunshot wounds to the head quadrupled in one of our major city's public hospitals.[1]

Physical therapists, long acknowledged for their accomplishments in restoration of function, must now pursue active roles in prevention and wellness in the health care system.

Jacqueline Montgomery, P.T.

REFERENCES

1. Stone JL, Fitzgerald L: Civilian gunshot wounds to the head. Neurosurg 33:770, 1993

Contents

1. **Acute Care and Prognostic Outcome** 1
   Kathleen M. Gill-Body and Marie Magliozzi Giorgetti

2. **Cognitive Rehabilitation** 33
   Katherine Sullivan

3. **Considerations in the Restoration of Motor Control** 55
   Beth Fisher and Susan Woll

4. **Management of Decreased ROM From Overactive Musculature or Heterotopic Ossification** 79
   DeAnna Anderson

5. **Evaluation and Management of Swallowing Dysfunction** 99
   Cynthia M. Zablotny

6. **Wheelchair Seating and Positioning** 117
   Mei Lee Chiu

7. **Orthotic Management of the Lower Extremity** 137
   Jan Utley and Cynthia Thomas

8. **Reconstructive Surgery for Residual Lower Extremity Deformities** 161
   Douglas E. Garland

9. **Reconstructive Surgery for Residual Upper Extremity Deformities** 179
   Douglas E. Garland

10. **Strategies for Community Integration** 199
    Mitchell Rosenthal and John F. O'Leary

Index 211

1 | Acute Care and Prognostic Outcome

Kathleen M. Gill-Body
Marie Magliozzi Giorgetti

THE CHALLENGE

The focus of this chapter is on physical therapy management of patients following a head injury in the acute hospital setting. Due to the nature and severity of the injuries often seen in these patients, physical therapy management will be discussed from the perspective of the various aspects of care required for these patients from the intensive care unit (ICU) to discharge from the hospital.

The primary focus of care for the head-injured patient in the acute care hospital is initially on survival and medical management with the goal of stabilizing the patient's condition and minimizing the effects of secondary complications. Of the estimated 2 million individuals who sustain a head injury each year in the United States, 500,000 sustain severe enough injuries to require hospitalization. Each year 75,000 to 100,000 individuals in the United States die as a result of a head injury. Of those who survive, it is estimated that 70,000 to 90,000 will suffer lifelong disabilities.[1] Recent improvements in survival and outcome appear related to advances in the initial medical management, making it critical that physical therapists treating head-injured patients in the acute setting have a current and thorough understanding of the common elements involved in the medical management. Therefore, we will review these common elements and incorporate this information, as well as fluctuating severity of patient illness, into the physical therapy assessment and intervention plan. We will outline a model for clinical decision making that specifically focuses on treatment planning based on the patient's level of awareness—a key predictor

1

of outcome[2] and therefore a very useful aid to treatment planning. Finally, information available regarding prognostic outcome will be included, as it relates to the patient's physical therapy management during the acute hospital stay.

Some unique challenges exist for the physical therapist (and other rehabilitation specialists) in the acute care setting that deserve special mention and consideration in a discussion of the head-injured patient. Often there are severe constraints on the amount of time available in which to evaluate or treat the patient due to the need for other care providers to have access to the patient and the patient's inability to tolerate prolonged procedures or interactions. Thus, the physical therapist must have a focused plan of care for each patient that is well communicated and integrated with the needs of the other care providers as well as those of the patient. Building or maintaining a team approach to the patient's care will greatly aid everyone's efforts. Initially the focus may be on the medical management of the patient and the functional or rehabilitation perspective may be omitted. Frequently there may be less emphasis or knowledge among team members about the secondary complications of head injury that are less life threatening but related to eventual functional outcome, such as joint contractures and muscle shortening, which may interfere with standing and walking. The physical therapist is key, in such a scenario, in identifying potential complications and developing an intervention program that is recognized and integrated into the patient's care by all team members.

EVALUATION OF THE PATIENT

Medical Record Review

The physical therapy evaluation of the patient begins with a review of the medical record. Specific attention is paid to the type and nature of the injury, level of consciousness, the extent and location of the trauma (both craniocerebral and throughout the body) and indicators of the extent of brain damage present. These can often be detected by noting the events that evolve, tests performed and their results, and the intervention needed during the course of the patient's initial hospital stay. Using this information, the physical therapist can often predict the possible impairments and consequences that may be present before even meeting the patient and thus focus the initial screening and evaluation procedures. Such a model for analyzing patients with neurologic dysfunction and planning evaluation and treatment procedures has been described by Schenkman and Butler.[3] Using their terminology, a *direct effect* of nervous system pathology means an impairment that results from the nervous system insult itself, while *indirect effects* involve pathology and impairments that occur in systems other than the nervous system. Impairments that have multiple underlying causes (some of which are direct and others indirect) are denoted as *composite effects of pathology*. As an example, if a patient presents after a motor vehicle accident with a closed head injury with diffuse axonal injury, it can be anticipated that the patient may have impairments in cognition and motor control related to the direct effects of this neuroanatomic pathology. If the patient requires mechanical ventilation, it can be anticipated that impairments in cardiopulmonary function will exist. Endurance for activity (if movement or activity is allowed or present) will likely be limited. The patient's ability to communicate will also be affected. Finally, in the presence of abnormally high muscle tone and a low level of consciousness, musculoskeletal impairments (such as abnormal alignment, joint contractures, and/or abnormal muscle length) can be identified as potential secondary effects of the neurologic insult.[4] The integration of this information allows the physical therapist to identify the most important areas in which to concentrate the initial evaluation within the context of the patient's overall medical status.

Other critical information to obtain from the medical record are the patient's laboratory values, vital signs, and medications. The vital sign flow sheet, commonly used in neurologic ICUs, can be reviewed to help determine the patient's ability to tolerate physical therapy intervention (Fig. 1-1). A list of medications commonly used in the neurologic ICU and their indications for use are given in Table 1-1.[5] Laboratory values and physiologic state may often be monitored through the use of specific monitoring devices in the acute care environment (particularly in the ICU) and are reviewed below. Specific contraindications to movement or position change are particularly important and will be noted below when pertinent to specific procedures and monitoring devices. Diagnostic studies or other procedures that the patient has undergone or that are scheduled to occur must be noted and their relevance to the patient's status understood. Review of the nursing and physician progress notes will provide a picture of the patient's condition since admission and allow any fluctuations or changes in status to be detected by the physical therapist. Finally, information regarding the patient's home and social situation should be noted so as to gain an understanding of the patient as an individual and to identify family members who may possibly be involved in the physical therapy program. This information will be particularly helpful during discharge planning from the acute care hospital.

Patient Observation

Upon examining the patient, it is important to note the patient's body position and presence of observable movements. In addition, the use of invasive lines, tubes, and monitoring devices must be noted and understood. Commonly seen equipment and devices as well as their associated indications for use and implications for physical therapy management are reviewed below.

Airway Management

Depending on the nature and extent of the injury from the direct or indirect effects of the trauma, the head-injured patient may be initially intubated to allow airway protection, maintain adequate oxygenation, and permit effective

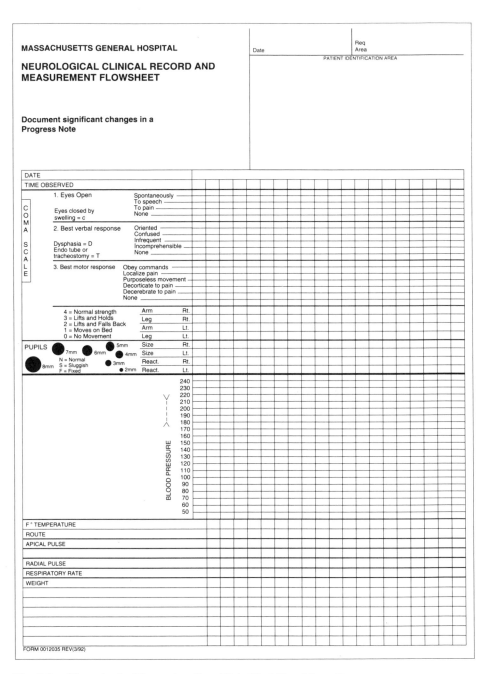

Fig. 1-1. Neurological Intensive Care Unit Vital Sign Flow Sheet used to monitor level of consciousness, pupil reactivity and size, blood pressure, temperature, heart rate, respiratory rate and weight. (Reprinted with permission of the Massachusetts General Hospital Neuroscience Nursing Service.)

Table 1-1. Common Medications in the Neurologic ICU

Name	Action	Indication
Ativan/lorazepam	Depresses CNS esp. limbic/ reticular activating system	Anxiety disorders, preanesthetic
Didronel/etidronate disodium	Inhibits bone formation	Heterotopic ossification
Dilantin/phenytoin	Anticonvulsant, antiarrhythmic	Psychomotor seizures, ventricular arrhythmia
Haldol/haloperidol	Antipsychotic, depresses RAS	Psychotic disorders, severe behavior problems
Inderal/propranolol	Antiarrhythmic, beta 1 and 2 blocker	Angina, arrhythmias, hypertension
Xylocaine/lidocaine	Antiarrhythmic	V-tach/multifocal PVCs
Lioresal/baclofen	Inhibits mono/polysynaptic reflexes	Relieves spasms, clonus, muscle rigidity
Mannitol	Osmotic diuretic	Increased ICP
Dolophine/methadone	Narcotic analgesic suppressant	Analgesic, weaning of drug withdrawal
Metubine/metocurine iodide (half-life, 3–4 h)	Nondepolarizing neuromuscular blockers	Respiratory/central nervous system control
Norcuron/vecuronium bromide (half-life, <1 h)		
Pavulon/pancuronium bromide		
Nembutal/pentobarbital (half-life, 3–6 h)	Depresses CNS	Preanesthetic medication, sedation, hypnotic
Pentothal/thiopental (short half-life, <15 min)	Depresses CNS	Anesthetic, no analgesia, anticonvulsant, hypnotic
Phenobarbital	Depresses CNS	Sedation, anxiety
Sublimaze/fentanyl	Narcotic, CNS opiate receptors	Short duration, <30 min
Valium/diazepam	Alters subcortical neurotransmission	Anxiety, hypertonicity

(From Murdock,[5] with permission.)

access for suctioning of pulmonary secretions. Tracheal intubation is generally achieved through one of three main approaches: orotracheal intubation, nasotracheal intubation, and tracheostomy. The first two are both achieved through the use of an endotracheal tube. A tracheostomy involves either laryngeal or tracheal intubation.

In the presence of an endotracheal tube, movements of the cervical region are generally avoided or performed minimally because of the potential for the tube to dislodge or cause injury to the walls of the trachea. There are no contraindications to movement in patients with tracheostomies.

For the nonintubated patient, nasal and oral airways are often maintained through the use of either soft plastic tubes (nasal airway) or a plastic curved airway (oral airway). This allows suctioning to occur as needed and helps to maintain an open airway. There are no contraindications to movement in patients with nasal or oral airways.

Chest Tubes

Chest tubes may be used in patients who have a pneumo- or hemothorax. The most common cause of these conditions is direct trauma to the chest wall. The implications for physical therapy management are that the drainage device must be kept below the level of the chest at all times and upper extremity and trunk movements may be limited due to the placement of the chest tube. Careful observation of the tube insertion site will allow the physical therapist to determine which particular movements (if any) place tension on the site in the unconscious, nonverbal, or confused patient. Such movements should be avoided. In the communicative patient, pain or discomfort should be used as an additional guiding factor.

Nutritional Management

Nasogastric or gastric feeding tubes may be used in patients who are unable to chew and swallow because of decreased awareness or consciousness, dysphagia, or facial trauma. If a nasogastric tube is present, the head of the bed is generally kept elevated to 25 to 30° to prevent aspiration during and after feeding. When feeding is not occurring, there are no specific precautions relating to movement and these tubes can often be disconnected from the supply bottle and carefully secured to allow the patient to be mobilized out of bed.

Peripheral Intravenous Lines

Peripheral intravenous (IV) lines are used to administer fluids and medications. There are generally no specific precautions for activity except to note that there is an adequate length of line for the patient to move without putting tension on the line. However, because the IV line may be located close to a joint in some patients, movement of certain joints or weight bearing during functional mobility may be contraindicated because of the potential for the line to become dislodged. This is particularly common at the wrist or elbow (less common at the ankle) and requires careful evaluation through close inspection with each patient. Often, a wrist splint is applied quite effectively to maintain the wrist joint in one position during such an IV line placement, thereby avoiding any extraneous movements of the wrist by the patient or caregivers.

Central Venous Catheters

Central venous pressure (CVP) catheters are utilized to monitor venous pressure, for the rapid administration of blood or fluid, for ongoing fluid management in the presence of a lack of adequate peripheral lines, and for the administration of long-term intravenous feeding. The anatomic location of the catheter placement determines which movements should be limited to avoid muscular stretching of the CVP insertion site. When subclavian or axillary CVP insertion sites are used, shoulder flexion or abduction beyond 90 to 100° is generally closely monitored to avoid tension on the insertion site. When external or internal jugular CVP insertion sites are used, minimal cervical movement is allowed.

Pulmonary Artery Lines

Pulmonary artery (PA) lines, more commonly known as Swan-Ganz catheters, are used to monitor myocardial function. PA lines are placed in similar body locations as CVP lines. Pulmonary artery, pulmonary capillary wedge, and central venous pressures are all monitored by the Swan-Ganz catheter. The precautions for movement depend on the placement of the PA line and are similar to those described for CVP lines.

Arterial Lines

Arterial lines are utilized to provide continuous systolic and diastolic blood pressure monitoring and to allow frequent blood samples to be drawn. Typical locations for arterial lines include the radial, dorsal pedal, axillary, brachial, and femoral areas. Movements of the extremity with an arterial line can be performed, but particular attention does have to be given to arterial lines located close to joints (as in the peripheral IV lines noted above) so that movements do not occlude the line. The number of repetitions and intensity of movements (or muscle contractions) may have to be limited in extremities with arterial lines to avoid dislodging the line, because dislodgement may lead to serious hemorrhage. The blood pressure transducer of the arterial line is aligned to be level with the patient's heart. Therefore, a change in the patient's bed height, limb position, or body position will often activate the alarm. Close communication and coordination with the nursing staff is essential so that the transducers can be adjusted or the alarm turned off temporarily during physical therapy intervention. An extremity with an arterial line is usually restrained when the patient is resting and left uncovered to facilitate close monitoring and easy access to the line.

Intracranial Pressure Monitors

Intracranial pressure (ICP) monitors are utilized in patients with raised intracranial pressure. This can occur due to cerebral edema or space-occupying lesions as a result of brain tissue injury. An ICP monitor is used to monitor accurately the intracranial pressure (normal range for ICP = 0 to 15 mmHg[6]), drain cerebrospinal fluid, and administer medications. Murdock provides a good overview of the four main types of ICP monitors commonly seen in the ICU: epidural sensors, subdural/subarachnoid devices, fiberoptic transducer-tipped devices, and intraventricular devices.[5] For epidural and subdural/subarachnoid devices (such as the Becker bolt[7]), a sensor in the ICP monitor (which is drilled through the cranium so that pressure in the epidural or subdural space is monitored) connects to a transducer which is located on an IV pole placed level to the patient's external auditory meatus (which approximates the lateral ventricle). The transducer gives a pressure reading that is displayed on a monitor at the patient's bedside, usually via a digital readout and graph. The angle of the head of the bed cannot be changed without careful coordination with the nursing staff when one is working with a patient with these types of ICP monitors, as this will change the level of the transducer, may produce incorrect readings, and may also change the pressure gradient intracranially. Fiberoptic transducer-tipped devices (such as the Camino sensor[8]) and intraventricular catheters monitor ICP via insertion of a transducer directly into the ventricles of the brain[9]; hence, there is no external transducer whose alignment must be adjusted if the patient's position changes. However, because intraventricular catheters also allow cerebrospinal fluid to be drained, it is important to ensure that the catheter is closed during position changes. Although a patient with an ICP bolt or catheter in place is in a critical medical state, physical therapy for gentle mobility and relaxation is indicated as long as the ICP values do not consistently increase with the exercise. For an individual patient, it is best to speak with the physician or nursing staff and determine what an acceptable ICP range for that patient is. If ICPs are consistently high for an individual patient (i.e., over 15 mmHg) even in the absence of physical therapy intervention, physical therapy intervention should be withheld until the pressures are lower. The patient's response to each evaluation procedure or treatment intervention must be carefully monitored. For example, if the patient exhibits decorticate or decerebrate posturing, the use of a foot board or foot splints may be contraindicated, as the ICP may rise higher when these devices are used.

Intermittent Pneumatic Calf-Compression Boots

Externally applied intermittent pneumatic compression boots are a commonly used intervention for the prevention of deep vein thromboses in patients who are on bed rest. The typical regime involves 24-hour use bilaterally with the exception of time spent during exercise or daily hygiene care. Placement of the air boot over the fibula head should be avoided to minimize the possible complication of peroneal nerve compression. Foot splints or other positioning devices (with the exception of a foot board on the bed) generally cannot be used in the presence of the pneumatic compression boots unless they are specifically designed to fit over the boots and not interfere with their function. This makes management of the patient with foot or ankle tightness a particular challenge for the physical therapist and is discussed below as a component of the treatment program.

Patient Position

Observation of the patient's resting position (particularly if the patient is initially in the ICU and options for body positioning are limited) will give useful information regarding potential areas that may need close evaluation by the physical therapist. Specifically, alignment of the limbs, trunk, and head should be noted to identify potential areas at risk for skin breakdown or contracture development. The patient's overall body positioning schedule with the nursing staff should also be noted.

Observation of Movement

The patient should initially be observed for the presence of spontaneous movements and they should be carefully noted. Spontaneous movements, if present, can appear to be purposeful or nonpurposeful volitional movement, automatic movement, or reflexive movement.[10] These categories of movement are described thoroughly below as their accurate identification is critical to assessing the patient's motor behavior and overall level of consciousness and cognition.

CLINICAL EVALUATION

Once the medical chart is thoroughly reviewed and baseline information is known—in terms of the patient's neuroanatomic injury, past and current vital signs, type and timing of medications, overall medical/surgical management, and precautions/restrictions associated with that management—physical therapy evaluation can safely begin.

Pulmonary System

Impairments in the pulmonary system, either from direct trauma to the chest and associated organs or as a result of injury to the neural areas controlling respiration, must be evaluated so as to treat and/or prevent the development of pulmonary complications. Cardiopulmonary physical therapy evaluation is critical as early as the first day postinjury because of the potentially life-threatening sequelae that can result from complications.[9] Evaluation consists of the following areas:

1. Inspection, including observation of breathing pattern and rate, use of accessory musculature, the patient's color and trophic changes in the skin and nail beds
2. Lung auscultation and cough evaluation (depending on patient's level of consciousness)

3. Evaluation of rib cage integrity and movement
4. Muscle tone evaluation in the upper body (neck, shoulder, trunk)
5. Interpretation of chest x-ray, ECG, and vital signs reports, arterial blood gas levels, ventilator settings, and ventilator weaning schedules (if applicable).[11,12]

Once these data are collected, specific treatment techniques can be utilized for effective pulmonary management.

Other impairments from the craniocerebral trauma can be divided into two broad categories: cognition and motor control.

Cognition

Cognitive evaluation is the first crucial step in evaluating a patient's ability to interact with other individuals and the environment. The term *cognition* can have a broad range of meanings, including a general level of arousal, the ability to follow commands, orientation to the environment, safety awareness, and judgment. Two cognitive function scales that can be used in the acute care setting are discussed below: the Glasgow Coma or Responsiveness Scale (GCS)[13] and the Ranchos Los Amigos Levels of Cognitive Functioning Scale (LOC).[14]

Glasgow Coma Scale

The GCS is an injury severity scale that measures changes in level of consciousness, which are considered the earliest signs of neurologic deterioration and/or improvement.[13] Consciousness is said to be related to the following three areas: eye opening (E); motor response (M); and verbal response (V). Each area is given several qualitative descriptors with a numerical value attached to each one. The sum of all three areas (E + M + V) equals the GCS score (Table 1-2). The range of possible scores is between 3 and 15. According to Jennett and Teasdale, the definition of *coma* is a GCS score of 8 or less. Qualitatively, they define coma as "not opening eyes, not obeying commands, and not uttering words."[13]

The GCS is a reliable tool to monitor neurologic change.[13] During evaluation, the best response is recorded for each area. When a GCS assessment is being performed, responses in each category to voluntary requests score higher than responses elicited by noxious stimuli. For example, a patient can initially be asked to flex his hip and knee; if the patient follows the verbal command, he will perform the requested limb movement and get a GCS score of 6 in the motor response category. If there is no response to the command, the therapist may apply a noxious stimulus, such as deep nail bed pressure to the hallux, and elicit a flexor withdrawal response. If so, the patient gets a GCS score of

Table 1-2. Glascow "Coma" or Responsiveness Scale

	spontaneous	E4
Eye opening	to speech	3
	to pain	2
	nil	1
	obeys	M6
	localizes	5
Best motor response	withdraws	4
	abnormal flexion	3
	extends	2
	nil	1
	oriented	V5
	confused conversation	4
Verbal response	inappropriate words	3
	incomprehensible sounds	2
	nil	1

EMV score or responsiveness sum 3 to 15

(From Jennett and Teasdale,[13] with permission.)

4 in the motor response category would be recorded. A similar noxious stimulus is used to elicit responses in the other two categories (eye opening and verbal response). When a noxious stimulus is used to attempt to elicit a response, the intensity of that stimulus may influence the reliability of the patient's response. Therefore, practice and consistency in applying noxious stimuli to patients is crucial.

The GCS score has been correlated with outcome.[15] Patients with lower scores (especially within 24 to 72 hours postinjury) have a poorer prognosis for recovery compared to patients with higher scores. In one study, GCS scores were measured within the first 24 hours postinjury and comparisons were made between the GCS scores and the percentage of patients within the score categories who achieved moderate to good recovery at 6 months postinjury. Moderate to good recovery was defined as disabled but independent and able to resume normal life even though there may be minor neurologic and psychological deficits.[2] Of patients with GCS scores equal to 3 or 4 out of 15, 7 percent had a moderate to good recovery; of those with GCS scores of 5 to 7 out of 15, 34 percent had a moderate to good recovery; of those with GCS scores of 8 to 10 out of 15, 68 percent had a moderate to good recovery; and 87 percent of patients with GCS scores of 11 or more out of 15 had a moderate to good recovery.[2]

Ranchos Los Amigos Levels of Cognitive Functioning Scale

The Ranchos Los Amigos scale (LOC) is commonly utilized by therapists in the rehabilitation setting.[14] The LOC has eight levels, and each level has qualitatively described behaviors associated with it (Table 1-3). The scale

Table 1-3. Levels of Cognitive Functioning

Level	Behaviors Typically Demonstrated
I.	No Response: Patient appears to be in a deep sleep and is completely unresponsive to any stimuli.
II.	Generalized Response: Patient reacts inconsistently and nonpurposefully to stimuli in a nonspecific manner. Responses are limited and often the same regardless of stimulus presented. Responses may be physiological changes, gross body movements, and/or vocalization.
III.	Localized Response: Patient reacts specifically but inconsistently to stimuli. Responses are directly related to the type of a stimulus presented. May follow simple commands in an inconsistent, delayed manner, such as closing eyes or squeezing hand.
IV.	Confused-Agitated: Patient is in heightened state of activity. Behavior is bizarre and non-purposeful relative to immediate environment. Does not discriminate among persons or objects; is unable to cooperate directly with treatment efforts. Verbalizations frequently are incoherent and/or inappropriate to the environment; confabulation may be present. Gross attention to environment is very brief; selective attention is often nonexistent. Patient lacks short-term and long-term recall.
V.	Confused, Inappropriate: Patient is able to respond to simple commands fairly consistently. However, with increased complexity of commands or lack of any external structure, responses are non-purposeful, random, or fragmented. Demonstrates gross attention to the environment, but is highly distractible and lacks ability to focus attention to a specific task. With structure, may be able to converse on a social-automatic level for short periods of time. Verbalization is oftern inappropriate and confabulatory. Memory is severely impaired, often shows inappropriate use of objects; may perform previously learned tasks with structure but is unable to learn new information.
VI.	Confused-Appropriate: Patient shows goal-directed behavior, but is dependent on external input for direction. Follows simple directions consistently and shows carry-over for re-learned tasks with little or no carry-over for new tasks. Responses may be incorrect due to memory problems but appropriate to the situation; past memories show more depth and detail than recent memory.
VII.	Automatic-Appropriate: Patient appears appropriate and oriented within hospital and home settings; goes through daily routine automatically, but frequently robot-like with minimal-to-absent confusion, but has shallow recall of activities. Shows carry-over for new learning, but at a decreased rate. With structure is able to initiate social or recreational activities; judgment remains impaired.
VIII.	Puposeful and Appropriate: Patient is able to recall and integrate past and recent events and is aware of and responsive to environment. Shows carry-over for new learning and needs no supervision once activities are learned. May continue to show a decreased ability relative to premorbid abilities, abstract reasoning, tolerance for stress, and judgment in emergencies or unusual circumstances.

(From Malkmus[59] with permission.)

ranges from no response to any stimulus to purposeful and appropriate behavior. The level of cognitive function is determined by patient observation across time under the following conditions: in various environments, at different times of the day, with graded stimuli, without manipulation of environmental stimuli, and with and without integration of physical activity. From these observations, a dominant level (rated from I to VIII) best describing the patient's behavior becomes apparent. However, a patient may also exhibit behaviors in two adjacent levels and hence be described in a range of levels.[14]

Relationship Between the GCS and LOC Scores

The relationship between the GCS score and the LOC level in patients with acute head injury has been examined through clinical observation with the following results:

GCS Score		LOC Level
3	=	I
4 to 8	=	II
9 to 15	=	III to VI

By studying these comparisons, one may deduce that the GCS may be a more sensitive tool than the LOC to monitor neurologic changes with patients in coma. The highest score achievable on the GCS, however, does not indicate normalcy in behavior; therefore, the LOC scale may give more meaningful information as the patient emerges from coma. By using these two scales simultaneously in the acute care setting, one can obtain a more complete clinical picture of the patient from a combined cognitive/behavioral standpoint.

Reliable measurement of cognition via these two scales is dependent on the assumption that cognitive dysfunction is a direct effect of the neuroanatomic trauma. Caution must be taken to integrate other factors that may affect cognition, such as sedation level by chemical means, sleep deprivation, metabolic imbalances, and hyperthermic state.

Motor Control

Motor control evaluation is the other primary area that requires careful attention from the physical therapist during acute care hospitalization. In this category are included such components as musculoskeletal evaluation, muscle tone evaluation, and motor output evaluation.

Musculoskeletal Evaluation

Prevention of musculoskeletal impairments is a key goal for the physical therapist in all phases of rehabilitation but especially during the acute care phase, when the patient may have cognitive, motor, orthopedic and/or medical-surgical restrictions preventing movement of one or more body parts. Yarkony and Sahgal report that 84 percent of patients transferred to rehabilitation facilities following craniocerebral trauma had already developed contractures.[16] Musculoskeletal impairments can include abnormal joint alignment, causing pain and restriction of joint movement, and/or decreased muscle length, causing a decrease in joint or total limb movement. The potential for developing musculoskeletal impairments in patients with head injury may stem from impairments in tone that lead to static posturing of one or more limbs. In addition, in a certain percentage of patients with head injury, the presence of abnormal postural tone may coexist with the development of heterotopic bone ossification. Heterotopic bone ossification is the ectopic appearance of bone in soft tissues, particularly in periarticular locations; it results in pain and decreased range of motion (ROM).[17] Another factor associated with the development of musculoskeletal impairments is weakness, which causes either a muscle imbalance across a joint or abnormal positioning of a joint. In addition, cognitive impairments associated with no other motor control problem may lead to musculoskeletal deformity if the limbs are not moved through an ROM on a regular basis. Musculoskeletal impairments that occur in the patient with acute head injury are secondary or indirect effects of the craniocerebral trauma. Direct effects of trauma on the musculoskeletal system, such as soft tissue and orthopedic injuries, may be associated with craniocerebral trauma and may further complicate the physical therapy management of the musculoskeletal impairments.

A quality assurance study initiated in 1989 at Massachusetts General Hospital's Physical Therapy Department monitored joint ROM outcome in patients with central nervous system lesions.[18] A sample of 18 patients admitted with a diagnosis of closed head injury were studied over the course of 3 years. Of these 18 patients, 56 percent ($N = 10$) exhibited ROM problems at the time of discharge from the acute care setting, with deficits present in the ankle joint (80 percent), elbow joint (70 percent), elbow and ankle (60 percent), and wrist/fingers (10 percent) (Table 1-4). All body areas restricted in ROM had concomitant increases in muscle tone. In addition, all patients with ROM deficits at discharge had febrile states associated with medical complications during the acute hospital stay. In contrast, although 100 percent of the patients who did not exhibit ROM deficits at discharge, had some tonal abnormalities, only 38 percent experienced febrile states associated with medical complications during the acute hospital stay. The reader is referred to Table 1-4 for comparison of other variables, including initial and discharge scores in GCS and LOC and length of stay (in days). Physical therapy treatment for all patients comprised a combination of approaches including splinting of the ankle, elbow, wrist, and fingers; bivalved casts for the ankle and elbow; air splints for the elbow; positioning programs; and both passive and active exercise and weight-bearing activities in sitting and standing as well as during functional activities. Whenever a joint limitation decreased or remained unchanged in a limited joint, a senior therapist was consulted and a change in the physical therapy program was implemented if considered appropriate.

These descriptive clinical data may suggest that patients with lower cognitive levels and/or medical complications associated with febrile states may be at higher risk for developing musculoskeletal impairments. Additionally, the greater length of stay for the patients who developed ROM deficits may indicate that a more complicated hospital course is associated with more musculoskeletal deficits even when a structured and monitored program aimed at minimizing

Table 1-4. Comparison of Patients Admitted to Massachusetts General Hospital (MGH) Diagnosed with Closed Head Injury Who Were Discharged from MGH with and without ROM Deficits

Variables	Patients with ROM Deficits at Discharge (N = 10)	Patients without ROM Deficits at Discharge (N = 8)
Tone deficits	100%	100%
Febrile state	100%	38%
Initial GCS range (median)	3–10 (7)	6–15 (9)
Discharge GCS range (median)	10–15 (12)	9–15 (14.5)
Initial LOC range (median)	II–III (II)	II–IV (IV)
Discharge LOC range (median)	III–VI (IV)	II–VII (V)
Mean LOS in days (range)	42.8 (23–92)	32.4 (16–67)

Abbreviations: ROM, range of motion; GCS, Glasgow Coma Scale; LOC, Levels of Cognitive Functioning Scale; LOS, length of stay.

ROM deficits is ongoing. Larger sample sizes with more descriptive data on variables, including physical therapy treatment, must be investigated so that variables that are predictors of musculoskeletal deficits can be more clearly identified. When predictors are identified, physical therapy intervention can be specifically directed toward improved musculoskeletal outcomes.

Muscle Tone Evaluation

Muscle tone evaluation is another parameter that is important to the acute management of the patient with head injury because the abnormal resting tonus state of a limb may lead to the development of musculoskeletal impairments. Tone can be evaluated and defined as the resistance of a limb to quick passive movement,[19–21] and impairments in tone may be a direct effect of the craniocerebral trauma.[22] The results of tone evaluation should reveal whether tone is high, normal, or low throughout the body. Although important in evaluation, this information must be integrated with the other components of motor control and cognitive evaluations as well as the patient's overall medical management before treatment strategies are initiated. For example, a patient may have ICP monitoring in the intensive care unit with a diagnosis of diffuse axonal injury and cerebral edema. This patient may exhibit high tone in ankle plantar flexors and decreased ankle ROM during one physical therapy session. If treatment decisions were made based on that one session, the therapist might suggest splinting or casting of that ankle. However, it may be that for this patient high tone is only associated with high ICP readings. Once the ICP is medically managed or at another time during the day when the ICP may be lower, the plantar flexor tone and ankle range of motion may be normal. Therefore, this patient's fluctuations in tonal state may be directly attributed to changing cerebral dynamics. Effective treatment of the ICP via the medical team may decrease the chance of eventual musculoskeletal impairments. Communication with nursing, especially in the ICU, is vital in interpreting findings and then directing physical therapy intervention. If the relationship between high ICP and muscle tone were not detected, the therapist might have directed treatment toward a casting program to prevent adaptive shortening of ankle plantar flexors. This might have been an unnecessary treatment. Although the outcome of the casting program could have been positive it would have been difficult to say whether indeed the casting program produced the good outcome or perhaps homeostasis of the cerebral dynamics brought about the improvement. Alternately, casting could potentially have been harmful to the patient if intracranial pressure increased further in response to the intervention.

Motor Output Evaluation

Motor output evaluation may be highly influenced by the patient's cognitive impairment.[12] Motor behavior can be divided into reflexive and volitional (or voluntary) categories, with voluntary motor behaviors further subdivided into conscious and automatic components.[10]

Reflexive Motor Behaviors

Reflexive motor behaviors are defined as "obligatory responses to peripheral sensory stimuli."[10] For patients with lower levels of consciousness and those who show no movement response to request, this may be the only evaluative strategy available to examine motor output ability. Stimuli are applied to a patient, and clinical observations of the motor output are then made. Commonly, noxious stimuli such as sternal rub, deep nail bed pressure, nipple pinch, and/or Marie Foix stimulation[23] are used to elicit a reflexive motor response. These clinical observations are noted in terms of which extremities or part of the trunk moved, timing of movement, range of movement, quality of movement, and return of the limb to the resting state. The intensity of the sensory stimulation may dictate the production and intensity of motor output. In addition, continuous evaluation over time should utilize the same sensory stimulation for a reliable interpretation of the motor output response.

Common reflexive movement patterns seen in patients with head injuries are decorticate and decerebrate posturing.[22] Decerebrate posturing produces marked extensor rigidity involving all extremities, occasionally head extension, adduction of the legs, and pronation of the arms. In general the arms are extended, although they may be partially flexed. In contrast, decorticate posturing results in extension of the legs and marked flexion of the arms, wrists, and fingers with adduction of all four limbs. The acute flexor posture of the arms is a point of clinical difference between decorticate and decerebrate rigidity. There is controversy as to whether these postures are constant or transient and what stimuli elicit the responses. These patterns may occur either continually (as in a resting posture of decortication or decerebration) or intermittently (perhaps secondary to dynamic cerebral changes such as presence of blood, chemicals, anoxia, infection, and toxins in the area of the brain affected). In addition, sensory stimulation—either as part of the evaluation process (loud auditory stimuli, ROM, position change, etc.) or secondary to environmental conditions (i.e., fan used to decrease patient's perspiration but patient in decerebration because of hair follicle stimulation, which is noxious to the patient)—may be the causal agent in the production of abnormal motor patterns. Similarly, abnormal patterns of motor output may stem from irritations within the body (i.e., full bladder, febrile state, etc.), which may be complications secondary to the initial neural injury.[24] Care must be taken not to elicit decerebrate and decorticate posturing when ICP is unstable, since it is believed that these abnormal motor patterns produce increases in intrathoracic pressure, causing heightened ICP readings.[24]

Voluntary Motor Behaviors

Voluntary motor behaviors can be defined as "postures and movements that are initiated by the person's own decision to act."[10] Within the area of voluntary motor behaviors are conscious motor behaviors (those that "are carried out with deliberate attention and sensory feedback")[10] and automatic motor behaviors (those that "are carried out without conscious attention and presumed to be under the control of motor programs established by learning").[10]

During conscious motor behavior, the limb movement can be described as purposeful, either the effect of responding to a command or a motivation that is self-initiated toward a particular stimulus or target. Alternately, it can be described as nonpurposeful, as when spontaneous movement occurs in a limb but does not seem to have an apparent goal or target toward which it is moving. Purposeful conscious movement can be graded via standard manual muscle testing or can be qualitatively described. Nonpurposeful conscious movement can only be described qualitatively; however, by changing the patient's body position and observing the movement in different situations, one may be able to apply a gross muscle grade to the movement. The patient's ability to consistently perform conscious motor behavior in each session, specific limbs in which movement occurs, the range and speed in which movement takes place, and patient positioning during limb movement should all be noted. In addition, stimuli needed to facilitate a higher state of consciousness prior to voluntary movement practice should also be noted. For example, if a patient is showing minimal motor output response, stimuli to heighten awareness level can be applied to the patient such as a cold cloth to the face, gentle facial tapping, oral-motor stimulation, and/or vestibular stimulation (passive quick head rotations or repetitive total body rolling). Once the patient is aroused to a higher level, voluntary movement can be reevaluated to determine if an increased voluntary motor response is present.

Automatic motor behaviors can be observed during transitional movements, equilibrium reaction testing, and other situations that utilize more automatic pathways to produce movement output. For example, if the patient is attempting to assist with a transitional movement such as coming from side lying to the sitting position, one can observe if the patient automatically utilizes one or both upper extremities, demonstrates typical righting, and moves both lower limbs in a way to facilitate the movement transition. Alternately, the patient may be dependent, requiring full manual assist, or may need to be directed by verbal cues to facilitate the movement transition (Fig. 1-2). If the former occurs during the particular movement transition, the patient exhibits automatic motor behavior. Where the movement occurred, the timing of movement initiation, and descriptions of movement quality are important areas to note during automatic motor behavior evaluation.

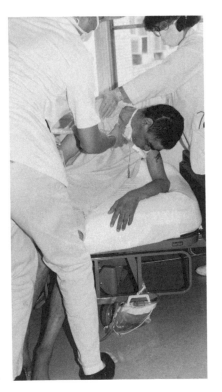 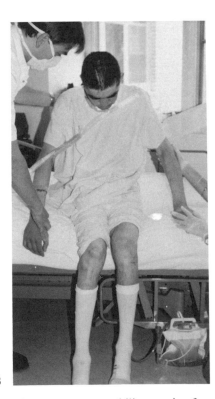

A   B

Fig. 1-2. Example of a patient with little automatic movement capability moving from side lying (**A**) to sitting (**B**). Note the lack of head righting, slumped trunk posture, and need for assistance (manual cues demonstrated here) to shift weight, use arms for support, and maintain sitting balance.

GOAL FORMULATION

Prognostic Indicators

Efforts have been made to predict outcome based on early clinical signs and symptoms to enable improved clinical decision making regarding which patients are most likely to benefit from medical and rehabilitation treatment. Age,[2] depth[2] and duration of coma,[25] neuropathology,[26] rate of recovery observed,[27] and duration of posttraumatic amnesia[28] are all related to eventual patient outcome (6 or more months postinjury). Access to a rehabilitation program has been shown to affect functional outcome, as demonstrated by Aronow[29] in a study comparing long-term (2-year) outcome in patients who received rehabilitation versus those without formal rehabilitation. Of these prognostic indicators, the depth and duration of coma are the most useful to the acute care physical therapist.

Treatment Goals

Once the pulmonary, cognitive, and motor control areas are evaluated and integrated with the patient's medical status, data interpretation can be performed to formulate appropriate goals for treatment. Guidelines for goal formulation and treatment based on the patient's cognitive status are presented in Table 1-5. These guidelines are useful to help guide clinical decision making for the acute patient with a head injury. Careful neurologic monitoring is imperative so that, as cognition and the ability to interact in active treatment improve, the focus of the patient's physical therapy treatment can be switched to a more

Table 1-5. Guidelines for Goal Formulation and Treatment Planning

Level of Consciousness	Treatment Goals	Focus of Treatment
GCS ≤ 8 →	Monitor neurologic status Prevent development of secondary impairments (pulmonary, skin, musculoskeletal)	Pulmonary care Positioning Range of motion/relaxation techniques Education to medical personnel and family Discharge planning
GCS > 8 →	Monitor neurologic status Prevent development of secondary impairments (pulmonary, skin, musculoskeletal) Facilitate patient progression	Pulmonary care Positioning Range of motion/relaxation techniques Movement facilitation (mobility progression) Education to patient, medical personnel, and family Discharge planning

Abbreviation: GCS, Glasgow Coma Scale.

functional and active level. In addition, constant monitoring of medical status is necessary so that goals are designed appropriately, according to both neurologic and medical status. For example, a patient may exhibit a GCS score of less than 8 but the level of consciousness may be lowered chemically secondary to the patient's high agitation level. Communication with nursing about timing of medication intake in coordination with physical therapy sessions will give the therapist a more realistic perspective of the patient's level of consciousness to then formulate appropriate goals for therapy. It is the therapist's role to tap into the highest level of the patient's neurologic function and facilitate functional gains whenever possible.

TREATMENT PLAN

This section will describe acute care treatment intervention in more specific terms, using the patient's cognitive level as a guide to specific treatment intervention.

Pulmonary Care

Pulmonary management is discussed first, since it is a critical part of the initial and ongoing care of the patient from a medical as well as functional standpoint and treatment strategies may not change dramatically for the patient with a low versus a high cognitive level.

Treatment strategies to decrease secretion retention may include techniques such as percussion, vibration, and shaking with suctioning if the patient's cough is not adequate to clear retained secretions or the patient has a low cognitive level.[9] Postural drainage in combination with these techniques is effective but may be contraindicated in the patient with unstable ICP. There is controversy in the literature concerning position changes and their exact effect on ICP, with some investigators reporting that Trendelenburg positioning may cause ICP increases compared to the head-up or head-flat positions.[9,30–32] Because of this, communication with the attending physician as well as nursing should be used to help guide decisions about the use of position changes for a specific patient. If a patient is on supplementary oxygen support, monitoring patient status with regard to blood gases and oxygen saturation levels during and after treatment is essential. The normal partial pressure of oxygen (PO_2) in the blood ranges from 85 to 100 mmHg, while normal oxygen saturation levels are between 95 and 100% as measured by an ear or finger oximeter.[12] Since various philosophies exist regarding the weaning process, it is important to know which one is guiding the care of a particular patient. For example, some patients will not tolerate any activity when the ventilator settings are lowered during the weaning process. Conversely, other patients will be able to incorporate activities during the weaning process. Education to nursing about the best bed positions for patients to decrease potential secretion development as well as for general tonal inhibition is important.[9,33] Early mobilization such as dangling, out of bed to a chair, and further functional progression should be encouraged as the patient's cognitive status allows nursing to facilitate improvements in pulmonary function.

Positioning

Segmental bed positioning strategies can incorporate external devices to align joints and/or inhibit tone in the head, trunk, and/or limbs.[9,17,19–20,33–36] Examples include the use of foot boards (Fig. 1-3), polypropylene splints (Fig. 1-4), and air splints[21] for upper and lower extremity positioning. In addition, foam wedges for head and shoulder alignment or foam abductor wedges for lower extremities can be very useful for maintaining good extremity alignment and preventing a loss in ROM (Fig. 1-5).

Use of inhibitory and serial casting deserves special attention, since appropriate use of these positioning devices can be extremely effective in preventing musculoskeletal impairments in the acute hospital setting. Several sources have encouraged early casting[4,37–40] and others have reported results of casting during the initial period postinjury.[9,39,41–44] Factors related to casting outcome, including patient selection criteria for initiation of casting,[37–38,41–42,45–46] type of cast applied (bivalved, nonbivalved, dropout),[9,37,39–44,46–47] casting materials used (plaster versus fiberglass),[37–38,40–43,45,48] duration of cast wear between changes,[49–51] and other adjunctive therapies used with cast wear[38,40,42,49,52–53] as they relate to the acute care environment have been previously reviewed by Giorgetti.[52] Use of nonbivalved casts may produce greater improvements in ROM with less skin irritation than bivalved casts,[11] perhaps due to the de-

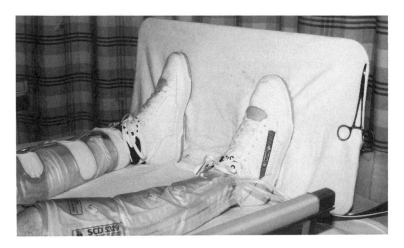

Fig. 1-3. Use of high-top sneakers and foot board on bed to maintain ankle joint alignment in a patient also wearing Venodyne air boots for prevention of deep vein thrombosis.

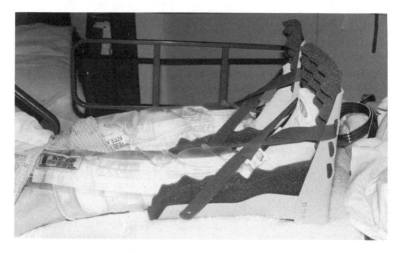

Fig. 1-4. Example of specially designed polypropylene foot splint that can be used over venodyne air boots to help maintain ankle joint alignment. Splint features include an adjustable angle at the ankle, heel cutout for skin relief, and optional derotation bar to align the entire lower extremity (not shown here) if needed.

creased variability in application that is involved in the use of bivalved casts by multiple caregivers. Although plaster has been advocated for casting material, the long drying time may not be appropriate for the acute care setting; use of fiberglass, which dries within 15 to 30 minutes, may be preferable, especially if the cast is wrapped with cotton material to prevent the cast from abrading the opposite limb. Casting is an adjunctive strategy to physical therapy treatment and should be incorporated with other activities such as positioning, weight bearing, and functional activities whenever possible.

Modalities applied to specific extremities with abnormal muscle tone or muscle length—such as ultrasound, hot/cold packs, biofeedback, electrical stimulation, and topical anesthetics—may be useful for inhibiting abnormal tone or reducing muscle contracture.[54,55] Nerve blocking agents and antispasticity medications may be additional effective adjuncts to treatment for patients who have increased muscle tone combined with progressive loss of range of motion.

A comprehensive positioning program can include bed positioning (side lying versus supine, with maintenance of head/trunk alignment and good extremity alignment) as well as total body positioning for the added benefit of total body tone inhibition via changing surface contacts, proprioceptive input, visual input, and vestibular stimulation.[17,33] Utilizing a foot board with the head of the bed in reverse Trendelenburg will bring the patient to a modified standing position with weight bearing on both limbs (Fig. 1-6). Using a portable tilt table will allow further elevation to the upright position and incorporate visual, vestibular, and proprioceptive input; potential benefits may include decreased muscle tone, increased awareness of the environment, a change in pressure areas on the skin and trunk, and increased lung expansion (Fig. 1-7).[56] Even

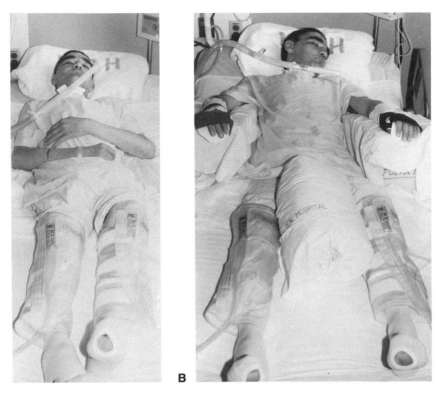

Fig. 1-5. Patient shown resting in bed without (**A**) and with (**B**) foam wedges, resting hand splints, and pillows applied for improved limb alignment.

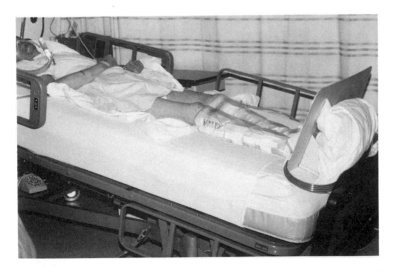

Fig. 1-6. Early weight bearing can be achieved with the use of a foot board and the head of the bed in reverse Trendelenburg for short periods during the day.

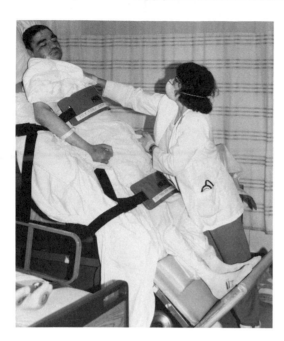

Fig. 1-7. Use of a portable tilt table to further advance a patient's tolerance to upright activity. The physical therapist is attempting to arouse the patient by applying a sternal rub and speaking to the patient.

the most dependent patient can be transferred from bed to chair with the use of good handling techniques and proper body mechanics. Maintaining normal head, trunk, and limb alignment out of bed in the chair is imperative as well; devices used in the bed for alignment and inhibition can also be used in the chair.[9,17,19–20,33,36] It is up to the physical therapist to develop treatment strategies for positioning that produce good outcomes and that can be easily transferred to nursing personnel for application on a daily schedule. The most elaborate positioning program will not be effective if it is not applied to the patient in the correct way and done consistently.

Range of Motion/Relaxation Techniques

Passive exercises to maintain limb and trunk mobility are an important component of treatment. Focusing on total body movement in the form of passive rolling from side to side or upper and lower trunk counterrotation may produce good ROM outcomes as well as tone inhibition. Nonnoxious stimuli (such as quick ice, vibration, or tapping) combined with assistive exercise can be used to facilitate muscle activation and limb movements. If nonnoxious stimulation does not produce the desired motor response, then noxious stimulation may be an alternative way to get active movement of a limb through a certain range, rather than just passively moving it.[57] Use of this reflexive movement strategy to elicit a motor response during treatment must be balanced with how the noxious stimuli affect body or limb tone, cognitive status, and overall physiologic state. Nonnoxious stimuli applied to all sensory organs in a daily structured regime are the basis of sensory stimulation programs. General goals of this approach are to increase input to the reticular activating system, structure interaction with the environment, and monitor the patient's neurologic recovery.[58] The usefulness of these programs has not yet been clearly demonstrated.

Movement Facilitation

Goals for the patient with a GCS score above 8 are similar to those just described (Fig. 1-2). In addition, the use of more active total body movements can now be integrated into treatment. Treatment progression can focus on utilizing voluntary active movements to command, more automatic movements, or a combination of both, depending on what motor output systems are available to the patient. Functional activities involving upper and lower extremity weight bearing should be incorporated into treatment strategies. Bedside activities can include balance activities using a Bobath ball (Fig. 1-8), poles (Fig. 1-9), bedside tables (Fig. 1-10), standing tables, and assistive devices. If the patient is allowed out of his room, mat activities incorporating upper and lower extremity weightbearing activities can be performed and patient can progress to functional gait activities.

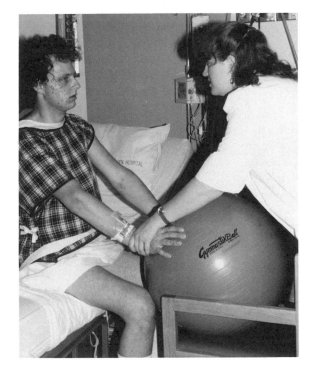

Fig. 1-8. Use of a Bobath ball at the bedside to help the patient weight shift forward and maintain his balance.

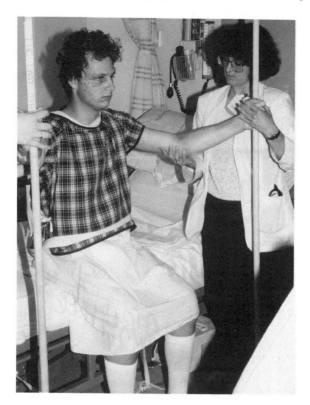

Fig. 1-9. Bilateral poles at the bedside can be used to assist the patient in regaining trunk control and alignment during sitting and standing activities.

DISCHARGE PLANNING

Contributing to the formulation of an effective discharge plan is the shared responsibility of all caregivers. The physical therapist is in the unique role of being the professional who can report the patient's functional deficits in objective terms. Therefore, it is important to state a professional opinion as to whether a patient's goals and potential for recovery can best be realized through a structured head injury inpatient program, an outpatient program, or the home environment. The ultimate discharge plan must address the availability of rehabilitation programs in a geographic area, the need for ongoing medical care, and the patient's health insurance coverage.

POTENTIAL OBSTACLES TO ACUTE CARE INTERVENTION

Variables such as medical acuity, lack of understanding of philosophy of rehabilitation care, environmental setting, treatment frequency, psychosocial status, and insurance limitations may challenge the acute care therapist and

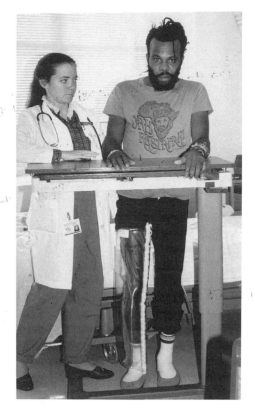

Fig. 1-10. Use of the bedside table combined with a lower extremity air splint to provide support to the lower limb during weight shifting and standing balance and activities.

possibly interfere with the effectiveness and outcome of the physical therapy intervention.

The patient's medical acuity may cause the patient to have various invasive lines, be chemically sedated, and have associated acute orthopedic and/or medical-surgical complications that can interfere with the implementation of various treatment strategies. The therapist must be aware of medical treatments associated with the need to sedate the patient chemically (i.e., for high ICP, patient agitation, or seizure activity), since they may dictate the length of time the patient may be in a somewhat unarousable state and may therefore change the goals and direction of intervention. Alternately, it may be that various environmental stimuli and approaches to behavior management may have to be adjusted to decrease agitation instead of controlling behavior chemically.

The lack of understanding of the benefit of early rehabilitation for the patient with a head injury may delay early physical therapy referral and possibly also delay intervention for the secondary sequelae of the head injury, such as pulmonary complications, contracture development, and skin breakdown. Strategies to facilitate early referral may include consistent attendance at social service rounds, in-service training for physicians and nurses, and consistent communication with nursing. In addition, meeting with each nurse manager or leader on a consistent basis may continue to strengthen a bond that facilitates a team spirit. Initiating patient care rounds in the neurologic ICU for the social service and nursing staff is one way to help facilitate early referrals and educate other health professionals about the role of physical therapy in the acute care setting. Delegating positioning programs and mobility exercises to nursing may require increased effort and education on the therapist's part, since a lack of experience in the execution of these treatment interventions may exist.

The environmental setting of the acute care hospital is such that there may, from the patient's perspective, be little routine to the day. In addition, sleep deprivation can easily occur secondary to the number of persons coming in and out of the patient's room daily. Lack of structure with many interruptions may disrupt recovery. Suggesting and implementing a consistent daily schedule for the patient may decrease patient irritation and facilitate behavioral recovery.

Delays in discharge planning, either because of psychosocial and/or insurance problems, may cause a patient to require changes in the treatment frequency and program as his or her functional and cognitive levels continue to change. It is up to the therapist to facilitate treatment program changes, delegate new activities to nursing and family (if available), and help the patient to progress in a timely fashion so that he or she is continually challenged from a rehabilitation standpoint.

CONCLUSIONS

The management of the head-injured patient in the acute hospital setting is a complex, challenging, and exciting area in which to practice physical therapy. The ultimate effectiveness of one's care is difficult to isolate and fully assess, as many patients continue to undergo neurologic improvements for months and receive physical therapy intervention in more than one setting. Intervention in the acute care setting that focuses on the critical elements outlined here will enable the physical therapist to establish a practical, holistic treatment program and minimize, to the extent that it is possible to do so, the secondary effects of the head injury and long-term disability.

REFERENCES

1. Statistics from Interagency Head Injury Task Force Report, February 1989. National Institute of Neurological Disorders and Stroke, National Institutes of Health, Bethesda, MD
2. Jennett B, Teasdale G, Braakman R: Prognosis of patients with severe head injury. Neurosurgery 4:283, 1979
3. Schenkman M, Butler R: A model for the multisystem evaluation, interpretation and treatment of individuals with neurologic dysfunction. Phys Ther 69:538, 1989
4. Leahy P: Equinus deformity in adults with severe traumatic brain injury: a pilot study examining incidence over time. Neurol Rep 14:16, 1990

5. Murdock KR: Physical therapy in the neurologic intensive care unit. Neurol Rep 16:17, 1992
6. McQuillan KA: Intracranial pressure monitoring: technical imperatives. AACN Clin Issues Crit Care Nursing 2:623, 1991
7. McKenna DM, Guanci MM: Intracranial pressure monitoring. p. 448. In: Puppe JM, Csete ME (eds): Manual of Intensive Care Medicine. Little, Brown, Boston, 1983
8. Hollingsworth-Fridlund P, Vos H, Daily EK: Use of fiber-optic pressure transducer for intracranial pressure measurements: a preliminary report. Heart Lung 17:111, 1988
9. Guanci MM: Increased intracranial pressure. p. 272. In: Hickey JV (ed): The Clinical Practice of Neurological and Neurosurgical Nursing. 3rd Ed. JB Lippincott, Philadelphia, 1992
10. Schenkman M: Physical therapy intervention for the ambulatory patient. p. 137. In: Turnbull GI (ed): Physical Therapy Management of Parkinson's Disease. Churchill Livingstone, New York, 1992
11. Boughton A, Ciesla N: Physical therapy management of the head-injured patient in the intensive care unit. Topics Acute Care Trauma Rehab 1:1, 1986
12. Cohen M, Michel TH: p. 9. In: Cardiopulmonary Symptoms in Physical Therapy Practice. Churchill Livingstone, New York, 1988
13. Jennett B, Teasdale G: Aspects of coma after severe head injury. Lancet 1:878, 1977
14. Hagen C, Malkmus D, Durham P et al: Levels of cognitive functioning. In: Professional Staff Association of the Ranchos Los Amigos Hospital Inc (eds): Rehabilitation of the Head Injured Adult: Comprehensive Physical Management. Downey, CA, 1980
15. Jennett B, Bond M: Assessment of outcome after severe brain damage: a practical scale. Lancet 1:480, 1975
16. Yarkony G, Sahgal V: Contractures: a major complication of craniocerebral trauma. Clin Orthop 219:93, 1987
17. Whyte J, Glenn MB: The care and rehabilitation of the patient in a persistent vegetative state. J Head Trauma Rehabil 1:39, 1986
18. Massachusetts General Hospital Physical Therapy Department: Joint range of motion monitor in patients with CNS lesions. MGH Quality Assurance Program, Boston, unpublished report, 1992
19. Carr J, Shepherd R: p. 99. Physiotherapy in Disorders of the Brain. Heinemann, London, 1979
20. Davies PM: p. 27. Steps to Follow. Springer-Verlag, New York, 1985
21. Johnstone M: p. 1. Restoration of Motor Function in the Stroke Patient. Churchill Livingstone, Edinburgh, 1983
22. Davis RA, Davis L: Decerebrate rigidity in humans. Neurosurgery 10:635, 1982
23. VanSant A: Traumatic head injury: an overview of physical therapy care. Part 1. APTA: Topics Neurol 11:1, 1990
24. Smith SL: Continuous intracranial pressure monitoring: implications and applications for critical care. Crit Care Nurse 4:42, 1983
25. Bricolo A, Turazzi S, Feriotti G et al: Prolonged post-traumatic unconsciousness: therapeutic assets and liabilities. J Neurosurg 52:625, 1980
26. Katz DI: Neuropathology and neurobehavioral recovery from closed head injury. J Head Trauma Rehabil 7:1, 1992

27. Gilchrist E, Wilkinson M: Some factors determining prognosis in young people with severe head injuries. Arch Neurol 36:355, 1979
28. Russell WR, Smith A: Post-traumatic amnesia in closed head injury. Arch Neurol 5:4, 1961
29. Aronow HV: Rehabilitation effectiveness with severe brain injury: translating research into policy. J Head Trauma Rehabil 2:24, 1987
30. Snyder M: Relation of nursing activities to increases in intracranial pressure. J Adv Nurs 8:273, 1983
31. Tsementzis SA, Harris P, Loizou LA: The effect of routine nursing care procedures on the ICP in severe head injuries. Acta Neurochirurg 65:153, 1982
32. Mitchell PH: Intracranial hypertension: implications of research for nursing care. J Neurosurg Nurs 12:145, 1989
33. Palmer M, Wyness MA: Positioning and handling: important considerations in the care of the severely head-injured patient. J Neurosci Nurs 20:42, 1988
34. Cardenas DD, Clawson DR: Management of lower extremity strength and function in traumatically brain-injured patients. J Head Trauma Rehabil 5:43, 1990
35. Edwards SM, Williams CL: Comprehensive treatment programs for severely disabled brain-injured patients. Clin Management 7:6, 1987
36. Shaw R: Persistent vegetative state: principles and techniques for seating and positioning. J Head Trauma Rehabil 1:31, 1986
37. Booth BJ, Doyle M, Montgomery J: Serial casting for the management of spasticity in the head injured adult. Phys Ther 63:1960, 1983
38. Ada L, Scott D: Use of inhibitory, weight-bearing plasters to increase movement in the presence of spasticity. Aust J Physiother 26:57, 1980
39. Barnard P, Dill H, Eldredge P, et al: Reduction of hypertonicity by early casting in a comatose head-injured individual. Phys Ther 64:1540, 1984
40. Zablotny C, Andric MF, Gowland C: Serial casting: clinical applications for the adult head-injured patient. J Head Trauma Rehabil 2:46, 1987
41. Sullivan T, Conine TA, Goodman M, Mackie T: Serial casting to prevent equinus in acute traumatic head injury. Physiother Can 40:346, 1988
42. Conine TA, Sullivan T, Mackie T, Goodman M: Effect of serial casting for the prevention of equinus in patients with acute head injury. Arch Phys Med Rehabil 712:310, 1990
43. King T: Plaster splinting as a means of reducing elbow flexor spasticity: a case study. Am J Occup Ther 36:671, 1982
44. Moore TJ, Barron J, Modlin P, Bean S: The use of tone-reducing casts to prevent joint contractures following severe head injury. J Head Trauma Rehabil 4:63, 1989
45. Cusick BD, Sussman MD: Short leg casts: their role in the management of cerebral palsy. Phys Occupat Ther Ped 2:93, 1982
46. Cusick BD: Serial Casts: Their Use in the Management of the Spasticity-Induced Foot Deformity. Words at Work, Kentucky, 1987
47. Leahy P: Precasting work sheet: an assessment tool. Phys Ther 68:72, 1988
48. Cherry DB, Weigand GM: Plaster drop-out casts as a dynamic means to reduce muscle contracture. Phys Ther 61:1601, 1981
49. Odeen I, Knutsson E: Evaluation of the effects of muscle stretch and weight load in patients with spastic paraplegia. Scand J Rehab Med 13:117, 1981
50. Gossman MR, Sahrmann SA, Rose SJ: Review of length-associated changes in muscle. Phys Ther 62:1799, 1982
51. Tabary JC, Tabary C, Tardieu C, et al: Physiological and structural changes in the

cat's soleus muscle due to immobilization at different lengths by plaster casts. J Physiol 224:231, 1972

52. Giorgetti MM: Serial and inhibitory casting: implications for acute care physical therapy management. Neurol Rep 17:18, 1993

53. Lehmkuhl LD, Thoi LL, Baize C, et al: Multimodality treatment of joint contractures in patients with severe brain injury: cost, effectiveness, and integration of therapies in the application of serial/inhibitive casts. J Head Trauma Rehabil 5:23, 1990

54. Cherry DB: Review of physical therapy alternatives for reducing muscle contracture. Phys Ther 60:877, 1980

55. Chan CWY: Some techniques for relief of spasticity and their physiological basis. Physiother Can 38:85, 1986

56. Richardson DLA: The use of the tilt table to effect passive tendo-Achilles stretch in a patient with head injury. Physiother Theor Pract 7:45, 1991

57. Umphred DA, McCormick GL: Classification of common facilitory and inhibitory treatment techniques: innate CNS responses to multi-input. p. 105. In: Umphred DA (ed): Neurological Rehabilitation. CV Mosby, St Louis, 1985

58. Radar MA, Alston JB, Ellis DW: Sensory stimulation of severely brain-injured patients. Brain Inj 3:141, 1989

59. Malkmus D: Integrating cognitive strategies into the physical therapy setting. Phys Ther 63:1958, 1983

60. Physicians' Desk Reference. Medical Economics Company Inc, Oradell, NJ, 1992

2 | Cognitive Rehabilitation

Katherine Sullivan

Recovery from brain injury is a fascinating and complex process. Brain injury rehabilitation begins at the moment of injury and continues to the level of maximal gains in functional outcomes. The health care environment of the 1990s reminds us that this process must be efficient and cost-effective as well as clinically effective. While the initial phases of rehabilitation are concerned with sustaining life and preventing secondary complications, each physical therapist involved in the recovery continuum must be a visionary, anticipating the long-term outcomes that serve as the measures of a return to a good-quality and productive life for the survivor of brain injury. The term *challenge* is frequently used to describe brain injury rehabilitation. The challenge for the physical therapist is to recognize that successful rehabilitation involves the interplay of both physical and cognitive factors within the imposed constraints of the health care environment.

Cognitive rehabilitation and physical rehabilitation are not aspects of a treatment program that stand alone. Yet how often have you heard a physical therapist proclaim, "There are no physical therapy goals; the patient is an independent ambulator." One of the primary purposes of this chapter is to encourage the therapist to look beyond the hospital, rehabilitation center, or home walls and develop treatment programs that maximize functional outcomes and improve the quality of life for the survivor of brain injury, decrease the burden of care for the involved family members, and satisfy the expectations of third-party payers. This chapter also suggests a framework for assessment that incorporates the interaction between cognitive, behavioral, and physical impairments. Finally, management strategies that focus on acquiring and sustaining skilled behaviors are discussed.

33

COGNITIVE PERSPECTIVES ON ASSESSMENT

The effectiveness of therapeutic interventions is a reflection of the basic assumptions we make as we define the problem, formulate goals, and determine treatment programs. It is imperative in brain injury rehabilitation that the clinician develop a plan of action reflecting long-term functional outcomes. The World Health Organization (WHO) has developed a classification system that can serve as an effective framework for strategizing a brain injury rehabilitation program.[1] This classification system describes the impact of illness at four levels.

1. *Pathology:* The underlying disease or diagnosis
2. *Impairment:* The immediate physiologic consequences or signs and symptoms
3. *Disability:* The functional consequences or abilities lost
4. *Handicap:* The social and societal consequences, including the freedoms lost or inability to resume previous life roles

Table 2-1 illustrates some of the common impairments and disabilities that contribute to the level of handicap for an individual after brain injury. Additional factors besides those considered a direct consequence of the disease process contribute to the level of handicap. Factors such as family support system, financial resources, and access to services are examples of elements that also affect the level of handicap. For example, an individual with medical benefits that include transitional living and vocational rehabilitation may have a greater likelihood of returning to work. Another example would be an individual with brain injury who requires 24-hour supervision; such a patient may be more likely to return to a home environment if he or she has a supportive family than if no family support is available.

Typically, physical therapists have focused on assessment and treatment directed at the impairment and disability levels. In particular, the emphasis has been the remediation of physical impairments and activities of daily living (ADL) such as bed mobility, transfers, and locomotion. However, if the physical therapist begins to formulate a treatment plan directed beyond the disability level to decreasing the level of handicap, the treatment focus takes on a substantially different intervention strategy.

Table 2-1. World Health Organization (WHO) Classification: Examples for Brain Injury

Impairments	Disability	Handicap
Paresis	Feeding	Return to life roles
Loss of selective movement control	Dressing	Ability to cope and adjust
Sensory loss	Transfers	Satisfaction with quality of life
Memory loss	Locomotion	Burden to caregiver
Perceptual deficits		Community integration
Aphasia		

DEFINING FUNCTIONAL OUTCOMES

What are the primary outcomes indicating a successful brain injury rehabilitation program? For the purposes of this chapter, successful rehabilitation outcomes are those that return the brain-injured individual to the least restrictive residential setting (i.e., home versus institutional care), decrease the burden of care on the primary caregivers, and allow that individual to engage in some productive activity, whether social or vocational. Obviously, accomplishing these outcomes is a multifaceted team effort. Together, the team, patient, and family determine the individual's abilities and limitations and the resources available that will result in the optimal functional outcomes. The role of the physical therapist includes incorporating physical skills into activities leading to decreasing levels of handicap. For example, the observation that the patient is an independent ambulator does not reflect the true level of handicap if the patient cannot use this physical ability to walk to complete a morning care routine without supervision.

The physical therapy assessment integrates physical, cognitive, and behavioral impairment measures provided by all team members, as well as the social and financial support realities, to identify functional outcomes leading to a decreased level of disability and handicap for the individual with brain injury. Approaching the assessment with this broadened perspective requires the therapist to reconsider the skills and abilities needed for the brain-injured individual to meet these functional outcomes. For example, a high school senior who has sustained a head injury and expects to return to school requires a level of ambulatory ability allowing him to walk substantial distances within the allotted 5 minutes between classes, find his way through the maze of crowded hallways, open his combination locker while holding his back pack, and so on. A physical therapy program preparing him for these skills and abilities is substantially unlike one that reports his ability to walk 150 feet independently.

COGNITIVE AND BEHAVIORAL IMPAIRMENTS

The neurobehavioral consequences of brain injury involves both cognitive and behavioral components. Cognitive impairments reflect the internal processes and deficits resulting from brain injury. Table 2-2 illustrates categories of cognitive deficits and examples of typical impairments within these categories.[2] As physical therapists, we can readily identify motor control and musculoskeletal impairments that contribute to overt movement dysfunction. However, cognitive processes involving arousal and attention, information processing capabilities, initiation, suppression, and direction of mental activity are all examples of essential cognitive function that converts movement into purposeful, goal-directed action. Therefore, movement dysfunction can be a result of both impaired physical and cognitive processes.

Cognitive processes are not directly observable; however, the observable behavior tells us something about the integrity of cognitive function. Behavioral

Table 2-2. Examples of Cognitive Impairments After Brain Injury

Cognitive deficits
    Confusion and disorientation
    Decreased short-term memory
    Decreased reasoning and problem-solving ability
    Delayed processing and responses
    Motor and verbal disinhibition
    Lack of initiation
    Concrete reasoning

Perceptual deficits
    Magnified sensation—visual, auditory, tactile
    Neglect or denial
    Visual-field deficit
    Right-left discrimination problems
    Pathfinding problems
    Delusions
    Hallucinations

Communication impairments
    Expressive aphasia
    Decreased understanding
    Delayed responses

Reactions to injury and disability
    Loss of control
    Frustration and anger
    Lack of insight

impairments are the observable external manifestations as the individual reacts and responds to the environment. One of the more difficult aspects of brain injury rehabilitation, which the clinician needs to understand and manage, are the aberrant behavioral manifestations occurring throughout the recovery process. Table 2-3 provides examples of aberrant behaviors exhibited during agitated or combative episodes.[2] The observable behavior of a brain-injured individual is directly related to the integrity of cognitive function.[3] The aberrant behaviors observed—such as confusion, combativeness, or restlessness—are reflections of the brain-injured individual's attempt to function in an external environment that poses challenges beyond his internal capacity. While these episodes can be both frightening and frustrating to the therapist, the therapist must remember that these behaviors are indicative of the brain damage and

Table 2-3. Agitated and Combative Behavioral Impairments

Wandering behavior: Erratic, unpredictable wandering away from assigned areas
Restless agitated behavior: Repetitive motor or verbal restlessness
Anxious-angry agitated behavior: Alarmed, disturbed, excited and uncooperative, unable to attend to instruction or cooperate with treatment; may become fearful, indicates loss of control progressing to combative behavior
Predictable combative behavior: Striking out in response to stimulation; disinhibited striking out
Unpredictable combative behavior: Unprovoked and directed striking out (hits, bites, kicks, etc.) potentially causing harm to self, other persons, or the environment
Runaway combative behavior: Combative behavior with eagerness to flee, escape, or leave premises

(Adapted from Klauber and Ward-McKinlay,[2] with permission.)

are not directed at the therapist in a personal manner. Guiding a brain-injured individual through a behavioral episode to learn to control a behavioral outburst is as much a part of the therapeutic program as providing exercise to learn to control movement.

The assessment of cognitive and behavioral impairments encompasses many clinical tools used by the various members of the rehabilitation team. Typically, specific cognitive assessments are not within the domain of the physical therapy evaluation. The intent of this chapter is not to review all of the various cognitive, behavioral, and perceptual measures; however, the physical therapist should be aware of these tests and the important information these measures provide.[4-6] The Glascow Coma Scale (GCS) described in Chapter 1, neuropsychological testing, speech and language assessments, visual-perceptual testing, and behavioral and social analyses are examples of clinical tools used to determine the level of cognitive and behavioral impairment. The physical therapist can use the information from other team members to provide a complete clinical picture reflecting the individual's true level of disability and handicap.

One clinical tool that deserves special mention is the Rancho Los Amigos Levels of Cognitive Function (LOC) (presented in Table 1-3 of Ch. 1).[7] The LOC is a behavioral scale which describes the progression of recovery as a function of cognitive recovery and concomitant behavioral changes. The LOC is a commonly used clinical tool to assess neurobehavioral impairment. This tool is particularly helpful for all professionals on the rehabilitation team, since cognitive-behavioral function can be readily integrated into the respective clinicians' treatment plans. The LOC provides a description of the relationship between cognition and behavior, identifies phases of cognitive-behavioral recovery after brain injury, and can be used to develop strategies for promoting recovery.[3]

DISABILITY AND HANDICAP

The physical therapist must be responsive to both the physical and cognitive impairments of the individual with brain injury and how these impairments interact to reflect the true level of disability and handicap. Leahy suggested a clinical model categorizing patients both cognitively and physically.[8] Individuals with brain injury are placed into one of three cognitive categories and one of three physical categories. The three cognitive categories are

1. Low: LOC I to III. Responses ranging from a limited response to stimuli that is nonpurposeful and inconsistent to some ability in responding to simple commands usually requiring multiple repetitions to produce the desired response.

2. Mid-level: LOC IV to VI. Confused, sometimes exhibiting agitated or aggressive behaviors; progressing to more consistent, purposeful, and goal-oriented behavior.

3. High: LOC VII to VIII. Some memory deficits present but more appropriate responses and some levels of functional independence; some difficulty in abstract reasoning.

The three physical categories are

1. Severely impaired: Dependent for most daily living skills due to physical disability.
2. Moderately impaired: Ambulatory with assistance or an assistive device or functional in a wheelchair.
3. Minimally impaired: Independent in ambulation but with high-level balance or coordination deficits.

The advantage of categorizing patients in this way is that it reflects the interplay of both physical and cognitive deficits in determining the level of disability and handicap. For example, an individual with minimal physical impairment but mid-level cognitive impairment may not be capable of living independently or resuming previous vocational or social roles. Physical therapists must be cognizant of the constellation of impairments that determines an individual's level of disability and handicap. Reflecting an individual's level of physical ability without reference to cognitive deficits may imply an erroneous level of functional independence. It also implies that the therapist must broaden his or her perspective on functional outcomes and the role he or she plays in functional training. For example, the physical therapist may report that an individual is independent in transferring from the bed to a wheelchair but requires moderate assistance to come from supine to sitting at the edge of the bed. What is the level of independence for waking up in the morning and completing toileting activities? Obviously, the true functional ability is only as great as the lowest level of ability within the task sequence, in this case moderate assistance. This example reflects a diversity of physical ability within a functional task sequence, but the analogy can also be made between varied physical and cognitive abilities. An individual who can independently ambulate around the home but is not able to call for assistance in an emergency is as dependent on supervision as the individual who knows enough to call but is physically unable.

In summary, the physical therapist's assessment must include an awareness of the cognitive factors contributing to the clinical picture of brain injury. While the physical therapist is not the team member primarily responsible for the assessment of cognitive and behavioral impairments, it is the physical therapist's responsibility to reflect physical skill within the context of purposeful behavior resulting in successful and relevant functional outcomes. In order to provide a meaningful clinical assessment, accurate goal formulation and treatment planning includes consideration of the following:

1. Cognitive and behavioral impairments resulting from brain injury
2. Cognitive recovery process and the behavioral manifestations

3. Interplay of physical and cognitive impairments in determining the individual's disability and handicap

TREATMENT MANAGEMENT

Integration of physical and cognitive rehabilitation provides an exciting challenge for the physical therapist. The therapist must be aware that there are two levels of management that evolve over the course of recovery from brain injury. First, the period immediately following the initial injury includes the natural recovery process. Positive change in impairment is often reflective of spontaneous recovery. Intervention focusing on facilitating the recovery process would emphasize treatments directed at the impairment level. Second is the level of management focusing on the degree of disability and handicap given a set of impairments. Epidemiologic evidence suggests that the greater the number of impairments, the greater the level of disability.[9] Intervention at this level would be directed at maximizing functional outcomes by emphasizing treatments that decrease the level of disability and handicap.

A two-tiered treatment strategy (one tier focused at the impairment level, the other on maximizing functional outcome) is a common approach in physical therapy intervention. Since the focus of this chapter is on cognitive rehabilitation, this two-tiered approach will be described as behavioral treatment strategies and learning treatment strategies. Behavioral treatment strategies focus on the impairment level by designing interventions in terms of the recovery phases represented by the LOC. Learning treatment strategies focus on decreasing the level of disability and handicap by designing interventions that are responsive to the individual's ability to learn.

Behavioral Treatment Strategies

One of the treatment assumptions inherent in a behavioral treatment strategy is that cognitive recovery can be inferred from progressive behavioral changes. For the purposes of this chapter and because of its widespread acceptance in the clinic, the LOC will be the tool used to monitor patient response. The LOC for the brain-injured individual is the most representative response determined by observing the individual throughout the day and in varying environments. The input of all team members is essential for determining the most predominant behavioral characteristics and how patient behavior is affected, either positively or negatively, by treatment.[3] The overarching goal is to help the individual with brain injury to progress to a higher level of cognitive function through systematic and gradated stimulation and activity (Table 2-4). Several resources exist which provide specific therapeutic activities for the various levels of LOC.[3,5,10–12] The following section is not intended to provide specific activities but rather to offer an overall behavioral emphasis for low-, mid-,

Table 2-4. Behavior Treatment Strategies

LOC	Recovery Phase	Approach
I, II, III	Minimal response	Sensory stimulation
		Preventive maintenance
		Monitoring response to early mobilization
IV	Confused, agitated	Structured environment
		Directed activity
		Monitor response to stimulation
		Brief, frequent activity changes
V, VI	Confused	Structured environment
		Directed activity
		Consistent approach
		Complexity of tasks varied gradually
VII, VIII	Automatic	Reduced structure
		Greater self-monitoring
		Progressively challenging tasks

and high-level cognitive management in which a variety of discipline specific activities can be introduced.

Low-Level Cognitive Management

The low-level responsiveness of patients at LOC I, II, and III present an overwhelming clinical picture to most therapists. The decreased level of responsiveness is often correlated with severe physical impairments. Chapter 1 provides treatments aimed at preventing secondary complications from immobility or severe motor control deficits. The physical therapist's role in low-level cognitive management is to provide the individual with sensory stimulation in coordination with other team members. Sensory stimulation can take the form of stimulation of the primary senses—visual, auditory, tactile, and olfactory—or through kinesthetic stimulation by moving the patient. Once the patient is medically stable and able to assume upright postures, varying his or her positions from recumbent in bed to more upright in a wheelchair or on a tilt table can be effective in evoking varying responsiveness. The therapist can provide valuable information by conveying to other team members the patient's arousal and attention to various environmental or sensory changes.

Mid-Level Cognitive Management

The transition from minimal responsiveness to confusion is often characterized by agitation. The primary goal of treatment at this stage is to help the individual progress from the agitated phase to a higher level of cognitive function. This is the time when most physical therapists are very frustrated because the focus on physical remediation becomes a secondary priority to the need to guide the individual with brain injury through this cognitive phase. The therapist must support the team approach in getting the patient through this period.

Physical activities can be incorporated into the cognitive program if the therapist pays special attention to the situations that exacerbate or subdue an agitated episode.

The therapeutic approach at this level is most effective if the individual with brain injury can be placed in a structured environment. This can include an area with little distraction and activity, or one in which the patient has room to wander safely and release hyperactive physical energy (Fig. 2-1). Once a structured environment can be secured, brief, directed activity that makes minimal demands can be introduced. Since individuals at this stage are easily frustrated, it is most effective to change activities frequently, within the individual's tolerance. Ideally, a schedule with frequent, short treatment times interspersed throughout the day is most effective in providing the patient with constructive and therapeutic contact time. Unfortunately, the hospital environment—which itself is structured in terms of 30-minute and 1-hour treatments—is not always in harmony with the individual's needs. The rehabilitation team must take a collective look at the patient's individual schedule. It is tempting (and sometimes very appropriate) to schedule cotreatments with other team members, but it is also wise to consider the amount of unstructured time that results when

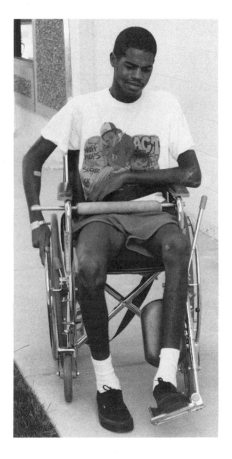

Fig. 2-1. Allowing the brain-injured individual to release hyperactive restless energy by providing a safe environment in which to wander.

these therapeutic choices are made. Prolonged periods of inactivity throughout the day can lead to boredom which, in and of itself, can induce agitated episodes.

Individuals at LOC V and VI continue to demonstrate severe cognitive deficits but with less frequent agitated outbursts. The primary cognitive impairments are severe memory deficits, high distractability, and limited ability to complete goal-directed behavior. The treatment approach at this level is to encourage successful performance by structuring the environment and activities to reinforce success. Compensatory strategies such as the use of memory books, a list of key functional goals, and repetition are used to help the individual organize his thoughts and actions. Consistency is a key factor to reinforce optimal performance. The confused patient should have a daily schedule, treatment setting, activities, instructions, and team of providers which are as consistent as possible from day to day. As cognitive function improves, task complexity can be varied by increasing sequence length or decreasing the rate of cues and feedback.

High-Level Cognitive Management

At this level, the individual with brain injury is more able to complete activities of daily living with relative independence. Cognitive deficits are more abstract, demonstrated by limited ability to generalize to novel situations or to react to subtle cues. Lack of insight or judgment is often a persistent cognitive problem in this phase. Treatment approaches that encourage problem solving ability in a range of tasks, particularly those preparing the individual for community reintegration, are appropriate. By reducing structure and expecting greater self-monitoring, the therapist exposes the brain-injured individual to situations forcing him or her to use higher-level cognitive function.

One of the key characteristics of LOC VII and VIII is a greater ability to learn than that demonstrated in previous phases. For this reason, brain-injured individuals at this level have a greater potential for cognitive growth, allowing for adaptation to home and community demands. It is this level, where treatment approaches must shift away from an impairment focus and more toward skill acquisition, that prepares the individual for assuming more meaningful life roles.

Learning Treatment Strategies

There is a key philosophic shift when one approaches a treatment program from a behavioral versus a learning approach. A behavioral strategy is essential in the early phases of rehabilitation, when the brain injury is evolving through the recovery process, and, correspondingly, through the various phases of the LOC. However, if therapeutic approaches are directed only toward the impairment level (i.e., dealing with memory or attention, monitoring response to environmental stimulation), then activities are not provided which develop the skills needed for optimal functional outcomes. A determination of the set of skills required will evolve from the interaction of cognitive and physical impairments and how these impairments affect the individual's ability to deal with self-care activities, degree of physical dependence on others, and psychosocial adaptability to engage in some socially relevant productive activity.[13] Inherent in the set of required skills is the capability to acquire skilled behavior.

What is skilled behavior for an individual with brain injury? As it is with anyone, it is the ability and skill to perform the tasks of daily life. Skill is the ability to consistently achieve a goal under a wide variety of conditions.[14] The ability to solve problems and generalize to novel situations reflects the individual's ability to learn. Learning ability is an individual's effectiveness in organizing available internal resources to generate and control solutions leading to meaningful interactions between the individual and the environment.

The ability to learn is often severely impaired in the individual with brain injury. Analysis of the LOC by learning ability suggests that the ability to learn is absent at LOC I to V, severely impaired at LOC VI, moderately impaired at LOC VII, and minimally impaired at LOC VIII.[7] It is important to note that the LOC provides general categories linking cognitive functions with behavioral manifestations. Other members of the rehabilitation team, particularly the neuropsychologist, provide specific clinical tests to determine learning ability. This information is a critical component in determining the individual's ability to generalize information to novel situations and in designing the most effective treatment strategies for enhancing skill acquisition. Conceivably, treatment approaches that are developed to improve skill acquisition should be structured in a way that accounts for the individual's ability to learn.

Learning versus Performance

As with other cognitive processes, learning is a cognitive process that is not directly observable, since learning is a reflection of internal processes and functions within the nervous system. Physical therapists are concerned with the learning of motor skills within functional tasks. Motor learning is a process associated with practice or experience, leading to relatively permanent changes in the ability to produce skilled actions.[15] Since learning is not directly observable, it is inferred when an individual demonstrates the ability to perform a functional task in a skillful manner from one situation to another.

Motor performance is the directly observable action; it is the level of skill in execution or how a person does a movement. When the therapist observes an individual with brain injury completing a functional task, performance is being observed. The distinction between performance and learning is important. Performance may vary from day to day due to fatigue, motivation, and emotional level. As will be discussed later, performance can be influenced by therapeutic interventions such as feedback and practice. However, it is the long-term changes in performance and the ability to generalize this performance to new situations that indicate whether learning has occurred.

Stages of Learning

The process of learning a motor skill involves three distinct phases.[16] The *cognitive* phase is the initial phase of learning involving the development of the execution program for the skill to be learned. During this phase, the learner makes frequent errors and performance is highly variable as the learner determines what to do. The learner is dependent on environmental cues, especially visual and verbal ones, to organize the movement. As errors decrease, the learner will begin to revert to other forms of feedback, such as kinesthetic cues, to correct the movement. This is the phase where a coach or therapist provide augmented feedback either verbally, visually, or tactilely to inform the learner of outcome errors (knowledge of results) or movement errors (knowledge of performance) in order to guide the motor response. Typically, the environment is stable, with few distractions, so the learner can focus on the most relevant movement information.

The next phase is the *associative* phase, where the learner shifts from what to do to how best to do it. This phase is characterized by less dependence on visual and verbal information, shifting toward greater awareness of kinesthetic or proprioceptive information. Learners are developing their own internal references of correctness, allowing for greater ability in assessing error-detection and consequences. Performance gains in this phase are more gradual compared to the previous phase, as the learner develops more consistency with less errors. The learner can be exposed to environmental distractions not present before.

After extended practice, the learner shifts into the *autonomous* phase. During this phase, performance is largely automatic, requiring minimal cognitive attention during skill execution. Tasks can be completed without interference from other external stimuli or other simultaneously occurring activities. At this phase, the learner is able to perform with minimal error and completes tasks with little effort.

As with most progression sequences, there is a fluidity between the phases, which shift depending upon task and condition. For example, driving a car is a skill most of us perform at the autonomous level. However, if the road becomes icy and you are not familiar with driving in this condition, your performance may decline to a cognitive level as your attention becomes highly focused on environmental cues in order to negotiate safely. An individual with brain injury will often demonstrate differences in performance based upon the environmental context. The ability to perform a transfer in a quiet, highly structured environment may differ substantially from the performance observed on the nursing unit with its multiple distractions. The level of performance proficiency (i.e., cognitive, associative, autonomous) is influenced by the nature of the task and the environmental context, which is reviewed in the next section.

MOTOR SKILL ACQUISITION

Motor skill is the ability of an individual to reliably achieve a goal through movement of the body. Skill acquisition is an interaction between the learner, the nature of the task, and the environmental context.[17] Effective training strategies, particularly those directed at improving learning, must account for the various processing capabilities inherent in task and environmental demands.

Tasks can be classified based upon their movement characteristics. One classification is to describe motor behavior as composed of discrete, serial, or continuous movements.[15] *Discrete movements* have a recognizable beginning and end. The movement can be quick, such as reaching to grasp an object or rising to standing from sitting, or longer, such as completing 10 repetitions of an exercise. In either case, task completion is defined as the distinct end of the movement. A discrete task does not represent a completed functional outcome but is a component or movement requirement of a task (Fig. 2-2).

Serial movements are discrete movements strung together and resulting in a meaningful functional outcome. Each discrete component, and the sequence of these components, is critical for successful performance. For example, brushing one's teeth is composed of a series of movements resulting in an action-oriented functional outcome.[17] Uncapping the toothpaste, squeezing it onto the toothbrush, bringing it to the mouth, and brushing the teeth are critical movement components in both their order and occurrence for successful task completion.

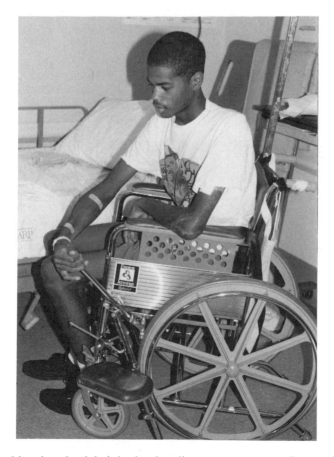

Fig. 2-2. Locking the wheelchair brakes is a discrete component of a transfer sequence.

Movements with no recognizable beginning or end are *continuous movements*. These movements continue until the action is arbitrarily stopped. Walking, steering a car, and pushing a wheelchair are examples of continuous movements. Continuous movements require a higher level of skill execution because they demand ongoing interaction with the environment to achieve success. Unlike serial tasks, continuous tasks cannot be identified by an array of subtasks strung together. Therefore, continuous movement would be considered more difficult, requiring characteristically different processing skills than those required for serial or discrete tasks.

Skills can also be classified by the predictability of the environment.[15] Since this can vary, skills are characterized along a continuum (Fig. 2-3). *Closed skills* are those occurring in the most predictable environment; therefore they would be considered the least difficult skills on the task continuum. An example of a closed skill is bowling. In bowling, the environment is always constant. Skilled performance is the ability to perform as consistently and accurately as possible to meet an established goal, which in this example is to score a strike. In closed skills, the skilled performer develops a repertoire of movements that are consistently and accurately performed from repetition to repetition.

Open skills are performed in an unpredictable environment. The individual must be capable of responding to an ever-changing environment. Skilled performance for open skills is the ability to predict or modify movement in response to environmental demands. The performer must develop a motor skill and be able to adapt this skill to changes in the environment. Walking on uneven terrain or crossing a busy street are examples of open skills, since performance is modified to meet environmental demands that vary from repetition to repetition.

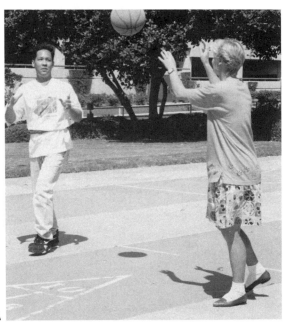

Fig. 2-3. (A–C) Activities using a ball require eye, hand, and limb coordination that emphasizes deficits at the impairment level. The activity pictured here requires responding to changes in the ball location yet takes place in a stable environment; therefore, it could be classified as midway on the closed-open skill continuum. *(Figure continues.)*

A

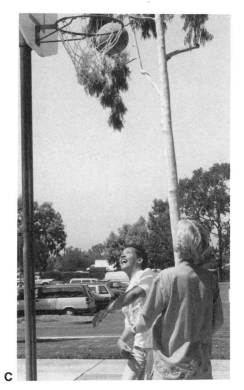

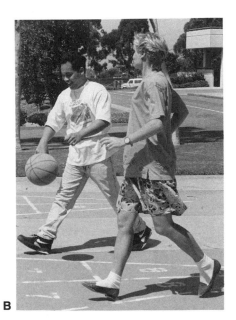

Fig. 2-3 *(Continued).*

Obviously, open skills are more difficult to learn and requiring more complex processing than closed skills.

While open and closed skills represent the extremes of a task continuum based on environmental demands, both levels of skill are required for proficiency in functional tasks. However, functional tasks should be considered on the more open-skilled end of the continuum, since the performer must develop consistent and accurate performance that is adaptable to environmental demands.[18] Most activities of daily living could be considered closed skills. For example, one's morning self-care routine is predictable in terms of environment and the customary sequence of events (toileting, showering, bathing, dressing). However, it is the responsiveness to unpredictable occurrences—such as the water turning unexpectedly hot in the shower or the phone ringing while you are brushing your teeth—that call for adaptability in this daily performance.

In summary, level of skill proficiency is highly related to task and environmental demands. Tasks that are not as complex and are performed in stable and predictable environments may appear to be performed proficiently at an associative or automatic level. However, as task complexity increases or environmental demands become more variable, a different level of skill proficiency may be observed. The therapist developing treatment strategies focusing on skill acquisition must be aware of the interplay of these various influences and how they affect motor performance.[19] Often, the therapeutic environment is structured to facilitate optimal performance. The therapist must listen carefully to reports from other team members who may convey levels of physical and cueing assistance in functional tasks that are more dependent than those observed by the therapist. The true level of skill is the performance observed in the home or on the nursing unit when the therapist is not there to structure the optimal performance environment.

FEEDBACK AND PRACTICE

Training procedures for both the coach developing an athlete or the therapist remediating an individual with brain injury share common features. The goals of training include the ability to sustain a high level of performance over time and to transfer this performance to related tasks and altered contexts.[20] Feedback and practice are two of the most powerful training variables influencing performance and learning. Research on nondisabled populations suggests that feedback and practice can be manipulated in such a way that performance gains are high during training, with detrimental effects on measures of learning such as retention and transfer tasks. The reader is directed to several references for greater depth in the multiple manipulations which involve practice and feedback.[20–25] For the purposes of this chapter, only a brief review of a feedback and practice application, which appears to be of potential significance to clinical populations, will be discussed and reviewed in the presentation of a clinical treatment model.

Feedback is information provided to learners informing them of the consequences of their actions and allowing for future error correction. Feedback can include knowledge of results (KR), which provides information about the outcome of the response in the environment, or it can be provided as knowledge of performance (KP), which provides information about the nature of the movement pattern. Such KR and KP are provided to the learner intrinsically via afferent information processed visually or kinesthetically through the learner's own afferent system or extrinsically as augmented feedback from an external source. Therapists provide augmented feedback when they use biofeedback devices or offer verbal, visual, or tactile cues about movement response or characteristics.

Feedback has a very powerful influence on performance. In the early phases of learning a skill, the need for feedback is high. Immediate, accurate, and frequent information provided during practice will result in performance improvement during a given session; this is important in early skill acquisition, as the learner begins to see how to do a movement or skill. However, recent evidence suggests that feedback has a strong guidance effect, steering the learner to the correct response and not forcing him or her to practice the retrieval and error-detection processes needed for learning.[26] In summary, feedback has advantages in early skill acquisition as the learner develops the capability to move or to understand the task. The disadvantages of feedback are that frequent feedback: (1) becomes part of the task, causing decrements in performance when it is removed; (2) blocks important information processing capabilities needed for retention and transfer; and (3) prevents the learner from developing error-detection capabilities.[20]

Feedback can be varied within a training session to maximize the beneficial effects and minimize the detrimental effects on learning. Continuous feedback is feedback provided during and after every task performance. Relative-frequency feedback is feedback provided through only a portion of practice trials within a session. For example, feedback provided after every other practice trial would have a relative frequency of 50 percent. A faded feedback schedule would be feedback provided on every trial during early practice and gradually withdrawn as practice continues. Although feedback provided frequently does result in better performance, relative-frequency feedback schedules, which prevent the learner from getting feedback on every trial, are better for long-term retention and generalization to other contexts.[24]

As with feedback, the scheduling of practice has a differential effect on performance versus learning. Structuring the practice session includes determining the tasks to be practiced and their order within the practice session. Imagine developing a practice schedule that is preparing an individual to complete the morning care routine independently. This routine involves several subtasks such as getting out of bed, walking to the bathroom, and getting dressed. Each of these tasks are composed of subtasks. For example, getting out of bed requires the ability to roll, to come from sidelying to sitting, and to rise from sitting to standing. Blocked practice is taking a task and practicing it repeatedly over a period of time. Random practice is interspersing the task throughout a multitask sequence. If the patient was having difficulty with sit-to-stand, a blocked practice session would have the patient repeatedly practice this component before introducing another. A random practice schedule would intersperse the practice of sit-to-stand throughout other tasks. The morning care routine is an example of a multiple task sequence where sit-to-stand could be randomly interspersed throughout the treatment session.

Research on practice suggests that random practice is more beneficial to learning than blocked practice.[21,25] As with relative-frequency feedback, random practice requires the learner to engage in higher information processing activities calling for the retrieval and use of previous information. If the solution to a problem is repeatedly practiced in a blocked manner, the learner does not engage in the problem solving and retrieval processes resulting in better generalization and functional carryover.

Caution must be taken when applying research on learning in normal individuals to individuals with cognitive and physical dysfunction. It is not assumed that the learning capabilities in individuals with damage to the central nervous system parallel those in individuals with intact nervous systems. In fact, brain-injured individuals present with known deficiencies in learning ability. However, the research on the performance/learning distinction is compelling enough to suggest that therapeutic interventions focusing on task, feedback, or practice strategies that facilitate performance may need to be modified to promote learning. Functional carryover in *multiple* environmental contexts is a better indicator of learning.

COGNITIVE REHABILITATION: WHAT DOES IT MEAN?

Cognitive rehabilitation implies the remediation of cognitive functions. But what are measures of improved cognitive function? The functions that become most relevant to the individual and his or her family members are the functions that reduce the level of disability and handicap. A clinical treatment approach that is sensitive to the interaction of cognitive and behavioral impairment—and how these impairments affect skill acquisition—may be more effective at identifying and developing the skills and abilities that increase the level of physical independence for brain injury survivors and decrease the burden of care on their family members. Factors affecting the level of care needed by an individual with brain injury include physical ability but, equally important, is the capability to perform self-care and vocational tasks consistently and in varied environmental contexts.

The cognitive and physical rehabilitation of the brain-injured survivor requires the knowledge and expertise of all team members. A team that can accurately assess physical, cognitive, and behavioral impairments, determine the social and financial resources available, and identify the most realistic functional and vocational outcomes will be most effective in meeting patient, family, and payer expectations. Table 2-5 presents a clinical model emphasizing learning principles as a framework for approaching the complex interaction of physical and cognitive deficits. One of the key features of this model is the identification of the brain injured individual's ability to learn. As discussed earlier, this requires the input of all team members, reflecting patient performance in clinical learning assessments and reports of patient performance in tasks throughout the day. The primary intervention strategy will be shaped by the brain-injured individual's ability to learn. If learning ability (i.e., ability to repeat performance over time in multiple environmental contexts) is poor, then treatment should focus on training performance. Training is the memorization of solutions which are generally nongeneralizable to novel situations.[14] If learning ability is good, then treatment strategies should be developed which incorporate motor learning principles.

Clinicians must assess learning ability as objectively and impartially as possible. Ideally, learning ability postinjury is an evolving process that improves as the recovery process continues. However, some brain-injured indi-

Table 2-5. Learning Treatment Stategies

Ability to Learn	
POOR	GOOD
Learning Environment	
Performance training	Motor learning
Closed skills; predictable environment	Open skills; changing environment
Discrete tasks; task components	Serial or continuous tasks; functional task sequences
Frequent feedback and cueing	Faded feedback
Blocked practice	Random practice

viduals sustain permanent leaning ability impairments (Table 2-6). For these individuals and their caregivers, the ability to participate in a task, such as a self-care activity, consistently from day to day under fixed environmental conditions and context may decrease the burden of care more significantly than protracted training in tasks that are irrelevant or beyond the individual's capacity. For example, a brain-injured individual may not have the ability to organize and complete her morning care routine, but if a family member can structure the morning routine consistently, she may be able to participate at a less dependent level. Performance training for the individual with poor learning ability would include determining the environment, tasks, and feedback that result in optimal performance. Since generalizability is not an expected outcome, tasks will tend to be closed skills with emphasis on task components rather than the ability to determine appropriate task sequences.

At the other end of the spectrum are brain-injured individuals with good learning ability. For these individuals, generalizing performance to new situations or changes in the environment are realistic goals. Ironically, therapeutic programs are structured to facilitate optimal performance and often do not provide the experiences and interventions that will lead to learning. Intervention that incorporates open skills in functional task sequences with attention to the scheduling of practice and feedback may prove to be more beneficial to skill learning. The therapist must be aware of the factors that influence the individual's performance level. For example, completing a task with the therapist in a structured therapy environment may result in performance at an associative or autonomous level. However, performance in a new environment with increased information processing demands may result in performance at a cognitive level. The therapist must observe performance in varied environments, modifying the task, feedback, and practice conditions according to the individual's phase of learning in that given situation. As skill becomes truly more autonomous, performance will become more consistent.

The therapist must also assess the cognitive judgment within the task. In Fig. 2-4, a man with brain injury performs a task that requires physical ability and high-level cognitive processing. This sequence also demonstrates his continued deficits in balance and judgment since he is using his leg on the oven door to stabilize himself. The most effective therapeutic program responds to the interaction of physical and cognitive aspects of a task.

The learning treatment model presented is derived from learning principles developed in studies of normal individuals, but little research deals with these principles in relation to brain-injured populations. Recovery from brain injury

Table 2-6. Learning Ability by LOC

LOC	Learning Ability
I to V	Unable to learn new information
VI	Shows carryover for relearned tasks with little or no carry-over for new tasks
VII	Show carryover for new learning but at a decreased rate
VIII	Shows carryover for new learning and needs no supervision once activities are learned

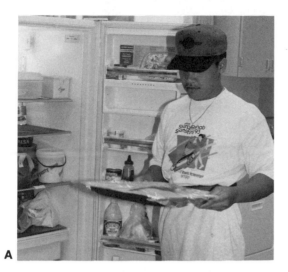

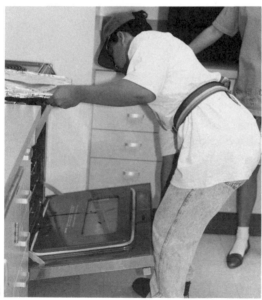

Fig. 2-4. (A–C) Having the patient engage in a functional activity such as meal preparation addresses deficits at the disability level. The therapist can assess physical ability, such as balance and coordination, within a task demanding cognitive processing, such as sequencing and problem solving. *(Figure continues.)*

appears to be correlated with changes in learning ability that affect cognition and the rate of information processing (Table 2-6). These processing abilities are the resources one calls upon to learn a new skill. The individual with brain injury may continue to engage in these processes but at a reduced rate; therefore the learning phase may be more extended at the cognitive and associative levels. Therapists must continuously monitor their programs to provide interventions that help the brain-injured individual to progress through the phases of learning.

The rehabilitation team must participate collectively in identifying the skills that will decrease the level of disability for the survivor of brain injury. The

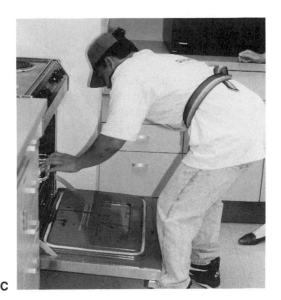

Fig. 2-4. *(Continued).* **C.** Note how the patient is stabilizing his leg on the oven door to improve his balance.

C

recovery process involves two phases[27]: medical treatment primarily directed at the impairment level, and reconnecting the individual with family and community. To facilitate this reconnection, treatment must shift from impairment-focused interventions toward those promoting skill acquisition in the tasks of everyday life.

REFERENCES

1. International Classification of Impairments, Disability and Handicaps. World Health Organization, Geneva, Switzerland, 1980
2. Klauber KW, Ward-McKinlay C: Managing behavior in the patient with traumatic brain injury. Topics Acute Care Trauma Rehabil 1:48, 1986
3. Malkmus D: Integrating cognitive strategies into the physical therapy setting. Phys Ther 63:1952, 1983
4. Thickman M, Ranseen JD: Personality changes associaed with head trauma: implications for rehabilitation specialists. Topics Acute Care Trauma Rehabil 1:32, 1986
5. Snyder Smith S: Traumatic head injuries. p. 249. In Umphred DA (ed): Neurological Rehabilitation. CV Mosby, St. Louis, 1985
6. Bouska MJ, Kauffman NA, Marcus SE: Disorders of the visual perceptual system. p. 552. In Umphred DA (ed): Neurological Rehabilitation. CV Mosby, St. Louis, 1985
7. Hagen C, Malkmus D, Durham P: Levels of cognitive functioning. In: Rehabilitation of the Head Injured Adult: Comprehensive Management. Rancho Los Amigos Hospital, Downey, CA, 1979
8. Leahy P: Head trauma in adults: problems, assessment and treatment. p. 247. In Lister MS (ed): Contemporary Management of Motor Control Problems: Proceed-

ings of the IISTEP Conference. Foundation for Physical Therapy, Alexandria, VA, 1991

9. Duncan PW: Stroke: physical therapy assessment and treatment. p. 209. In Lister MS (ed): Contemporary Management of Motor Control Problems: Proceedings of the IISETP Conference. Foundation for Physical Therapy, Alexandria, VA, 1991

10. Messa J: Overview of physical therapy management of patients with traumatic brain injury. Neurol Rep 14:9, 1990

11. Van Sant A: Traumatic head injury: an overview of physical therapy care: Part 1. APTA: Topics Neurol 11:1, 1990

12. Van Sant A: Traumatic head injury: an overview of physical therapy care: Part 2. APTA: Topics Neurol 12:1, 1990

13. Rappaport M, Hall KM, Hopkins K, et al: Disability rating scale for severe head trauma: coma to community. Arch Phys Med Rehabil 63:118, 1982

14. Higgins S: Motor skill acquisition. Phys Ther 71:123, 1991

15. Schmidt RA: Motor Control and Learning: A Behavioral Emphasis, Ed. 2. Human Kinetics, Champaign, IL, 1988

16. Fitts PM, Posner MI: Human Performance. Brooks/Cole, Belmont, CA, 1967

17. Gentile AM: Skill acquisition: action, movement, and neuromotor processes. p. 93. In Carr JH, Shepherd RB (eds): Movement Science Foundations for Physical Therapy in Rehabilitation. Aspen Publishers, Rockville, MD, 1987

18. Winstein CJ: Motor learning considerations in stroke rehabilitation. p. 109. In Duncan PW, Badke MB (eds): Stroke Rehabilitation: The Recovery of Motor Control. Yearbook Medical Publishers, Chicago, 1987

19. Barton LA, Sullivan Black K: Learning treatment strategies applied to stroke rehabilitation. p. 63. In Gordon WA (ed): Advances in Stroke Rehabilitation. Andover Medical Publishers, Boston, 1993

20. Schmidt RA, Bjork RA: New conceptualizations of practice: common principles in three paradigms suggest new concepts for training. Am Psychol Soc 3:207, 1992

21. Lee TD, Swanson LR, Hall AL: What is repeated in repetition? Effect of practice conditions on motor skill acquisition. Phys Ther 71:150, 1991

22. Schmidt RA: Motor learning principles for physical therapy. p. 49. In Lister MS (ed): Contemporary Management of Motor Control Problems: Proceedings of the IISTEP Conference. Foundation for Physical Therapy, Alexandria, VA, 1991

23. Winstein CJ: Designing practice for motor learning: clinical implications. p. 65. In Lister MS (ed): Contemporary Management of Motor Control Problems: Proceedings of the IISTEP Conference. Foundation for Physical Therapy, Alexandria, VA, 1991

24. Winstein CJ: Knowledge of results and motor learning: implications for physical therapy. Phys Ther 71:140, 1991

25. Chamberlain C, Lee T: Arranging practice conditions and designing practice. p. 231. In Singer RN, Murphy M, Tenant LK (eds): Handbook of Research on Sport Psychology. Macmillan, New York, 1993

26. Winstein CJ, Schmidt RA: Reduced frequency of knowledge of results enhances motor skill learning. J Exp Psych: Learn Mem Cog 16:677, 1990

27. Condeluci A: Brain injury rehabilitation: the need to bridge paradigms. Brain Inj 6: 543, 1992

3 | Considerations in the Restoration of Motor Control

Beth Fisher
Susan Woll

There is ample evidence in the physical therapy efficacy literature to suggest that techniques can be utilized to produce motor responses in the affected limbs of patients with brain lesions.[1-4] However, the critical issue is whether the patient develops the ability to incorporate use of the affected limbs in his or her daily existence. Evidence for this more crucial issue, although beginning to emerge, is scarce.[5] This, in part, has led to ever-increasing disillusion with the prospect of true restitution of motor function by physical therapy intervention. Indeed, it has sparked the current controversy as to whether the focus of rehabilitation should be solely on assisting the patient to develop compensatory strategies that allow for completion of basic functional tasks versus the retraining of skills in a manner promoting the use of the affected body segments and their incorporation into those skills.[6]

Driving one end of the argument are practical issues related to the ever-increasing limitations on the time available in which to render physical therapy services. The "push" then becomes one of making the patient functionally independent (by inpatient rehabilitation standards, i.e., transfers and household ambulation) as quickly as possible. On the other hand, basic science research with experimental animals suggests that a potential for recovery of function in the affected extremities does exist but may well, in fact, be eliminated if the animal is able to accomplish the task utilizing a compensatory strategy.[7-9] In other words, rather than being "lesion-driven," behavioral deficits result from what might be considered animal and human nature to automatically compensate and essentially take the path of least resistance. Thus, the very compensation eliminates the need to recover use of the affected body segments. Further, studies have suggested that perhaps the issue is not that the animal or human is unable to use the affected extremities following a peripheral or central nervous system lesion, but that they essentially make the "choice" not to so that they can more readily perform, albeit in a substitutive capacity, a functional task.[7-11] This then leads to what Taub calls a "learned nonuse syndrome."[9]

Clearly, there are compelling arguments on both sides of the controversy regarding compensation versus movement reeducation, but is it up to us to decide? As therapists are setting up "camps"—one group advocating function utilizing compensatory strategies, one group advocating optimizing recovery of function in the affected extremities—we must ask ourselves: "Has anyone bothered to consult the patient?" It is the contention of the authors that it is the responsibility of the therapist to lay out the options for the patient and the family and allow them to make the choice to either compensate for deficits or work on the elimination of deficits.

The patient must be informed that a good deal of recovery may in fact be possible and that it could be impeded by compensation. Currently, patients and families are told that almost all "spontaneous recovery" of function following a brain injury occurs within the first 6 months and virtually none after 1 year.[12] Rapid and spontaneous recovery of function may well occur within certain time frames, but the patient must know that, through extensive training and practice, substantial gains can be made over his or her *lifetime*. Patients must be informed that their early choices may affect this. For example, the longer the patient performs daily tasks without incorporating the affected extremities, the more likely it is that secondary changes in the musculoskeletal system (i.e., decreased mobility and force production) will develop and become primary problems to be overcome. The fact that, on average, brain-injured patients are in their twenties means that the possibility of acquiring new skills over a lifetime could amount to 50 years.

In addition, the issue for the therapist involved in treating the brain-injured patient need not be having to choose between functional training and promoting recovery. Functional tasks can be set up and practiced in a way that both promotes independence and encourages use of the affected segments. The authors support the position not only that recovery is possible but that therapists involved in the treatment of brain-injured patients should "expect" recovery and develop intervention strategies that prevent or at least minimize compensation for those patients whose choice it is to take this route.

This chapter, therefore, focuses on issues related to the restoration of functional use of the affected body segments within task-specific training. Both theoretical and practical concepts are presented to help therapists design treatment sessions for their brain-injured clients.

THE CONTROVERSY OVER COMPENSATION VERSUS MOVEMENT REEDUCATION

Normal, healthy individuals operate according to the following principle: "Most functional tasks can be achieved with a variety of movement patterns, but we tend to use the one that requires the least amount of energy and that is the most efficient melding on the many parts involved."[13] Brain-injured patients arrive at their patterns of movement according to similar principles. But if therapy is going to stress or challenge unused or affected limbs and affected neural systems, then therapists must counter this normal tendency.

The therapeutic community is starting to recognize that the behavioral deficits seen in the brain-injured patient are not just neuropathologic but are related to the propensity to compensate, do what is easier and less risky, and that movement abnormalities are perhaps physical and or biomechanical consequences of the patient's chosen movement strategies. The question that must be addressed is this: If a patient can achieve a goal utilizing a compensatory strategy, isn't that sufficient? In order to answer that question it is important to consider the upper limits of the strategy.

Normal movement is perhaps not an issue of specific and invariant movement patterns but relates more to one's ability to link numbers of behaviors together, do more than one thing at a time, and effectively perform tasks under a variety of environmental conditions. For example, a healthy individual does not simply move from sitting to standing. Such a person is able to progress from sitting to standing to gait as one continuous movement. Furthermore, the individual is capable of accomplishing those transitions regardless of the sitting surface and floor characteristics, while conversing or holding or manipulating objects, or with his or her attention directed at something that is entirely unrelated to the activity. The brain-injured patient, on the other hand, often operates in more "discrete packets of behavior," and is forced by his or her strategy to begin and end one movement before beginning the next. For example, after a brain injury, because of sensory and motor deficits, a patient may perceive his lower limb as incapable of supporting his body weight. Given this perception, his choice then—to maintain the body's center of mass posterior to the feet and aligned over the sound side while preparing to stand—should not be viewed as "abnormal" but as an entirely reasonable and sound compensation. The problem is not the automatic shift in control to the sound side but the profound limitation this choice has on outcome.

LeVere defines compensation as a substitutive process in which nothing is recovered but in which a new and sometimes grossly different behavior is acquired to attenuate behavioral deficiencies produced by the brain injury.[14] For example, the starting alignment of the patient described above commonly favors the following chain of events: The shift of the patient toward the sound side in a position of trunk flexion and pelvic posterior tilt induces a backward rotation of the pelvis on the involved side. The femur on that side abducts, creating a situation in which the knee is lateral to the foot, thus biasing the foot to assume a supinated posture. Maintaining his weight on the pelvis forces this patient to create momentum by rocking back and forth or pulling with the sound arm in order to propel himself off the seat. Once off the surface, the tibias are driven back in order to counterbalance the effect of a large portion of the body's center of mass ending up anterior to the new base of support, the feet. Strictly from the standpoint of the biomechanical constraints that exist, given the choice to maintain weight shifted back and to one side, movement pattern options in the lower extremities are limited. Essentially, the odds are stacked in favor of the patient demonstrating what has been described as an abnormal extensor pattern in the lower extremity, with the knee fully locked in extension and the foot supinated and out of weight bearing. The ''grossly different behavior'' the patient has utilized to attenuate behavioral deficiencies produced by the brain lesion has limited the outcome to only standing. Unable to attain a squat posture once off the surface, this person does not have the option of stopping part way up to pick up an object from the sitting surface or to proceed directly into the activity that prompted him to get up in the first place. A limited version of the former behavior has been achieved but is inadequate to meet the demands of a fast-paced, unpredictable environment such as a university or work setting.

THE INVESTMENT PRINCIPLE

Thus far, the argument is that to promote strategies for movement that incorporate the involved body segments, increase the patient's repertoire of movement options, and maximize potential for functional use of the involved extremities, compensation should be minimized. This is a somewhat overwhelming prospect in that the therapist is then asking the patient essentially to go *against* what would be the natural tendency to take the path of least resistance. Choosing to take the more difficult path is often complicated by the fact that the patient may initially experience a decline in task performance to learn the new strategy.

This concept is illustrated by what James Gordon calls ''the investment principle.''[15] In Figure 3-1, it can be seen that over time, and presumably with practice in utilizing a certain strategy for completing a task (old strategy), *performance* of the task will improve. If at a certain point in time a new strategy for the task is attempted (perhaps imposed on the performer by a coach, trainer, or therapist), there will be an initial decline in performance. This is most likely because the performer is unfamiliar with the new strategy. Over time, however, with continued practice of the new strategy, there is the potential for enhanced performance well beyond that afforded by the old strategy. The performer, at this point, has realized a ''greater return'' on the investment.

A person who decides to take tennis lessons after developing some skill with the sport may experience this phenomenon. Commonly, the initial instruction in how to hold the tennis racquet is unfamiliar, unlike what the person has done previously, and even awkward. That person, in fact, experiences a decline in ability to play the game. However, if the coach or trainer helps the person

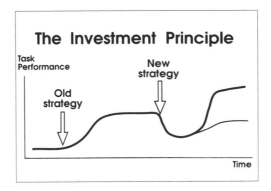

Fig. 3-1.   The investment principle. (Courtesy of James Gordon, 1992.)

experience that holding the racquet in that manner enables him or her to put greater force behind the ball and hit it with greater accuracy, then the benefit of the initial investment can be readily identified and will promote continued practice.

Clinical examples illustrating this concept are numerous. For example, patients with unilateral involvement often figure out that they can solve the problem of moving from sitting to standing by pushing or pulling with the intact upper extremity. The immediate goal of standing has been achieved, most likely in the only way the patient thought was possible, perhaps in the only way the patient feels safe. Goal attainment reinforces the strategy to the point that it becomes automatic for the patient to perform in this manner.

The therapist interested in promoting functional use of the involved limbs may recognize that this is a sound short-term solution to the problem of attaining a standing posture but, in fact, may eliminate the long-term possibility of enhanced control and strength of the involved arm and leg. The therapist therefore tries to encourage the patient, perhaps with manual and verbal guidance, to develop a strategy whereby weight is shifted forward and the patient pushes equally with both legs.

One could argue that a strategy such as this, in which the energy demands of the task are shared or divided throughout the whole body, is more efficient and therefore easier than using one or two limbs. However, not only is this initially more difficult for the patient but he may in fact experience a decline in his performance. He experiences that it takes him longer to perform the transition to standing. He has to think about what he is doing and has to coordinate the movement in a different way. What could possibly persuade this patient to make the investment?

For too long, therapists have relied on the idea that there should be compliance with the established physical therapy program because they are the most knowledgeable regarding the needs of the patient. A therapist trying to convince a patient of the need to develop an alternative strategy in performing a task might say the following: "Yes, I can see that you are able to get yourself to standing by pulling with your arm, but you really need to learn how to do that *this* way, or my way. Your way won't help your leg get stronger." Perhaps there has been too little attempt at providing an experience for the patient which substantiates the benefit of that alternative. In every treatment session, the patient must experience what it "buys him," what it affords him to work at practicing a more difficult strategy for a task and one which initially may entail a decline in task performance. The therapist must set up the possibility for the patient to be able to make a comparison between two outcomes, one of which is perceived as a favorable or more desirable outcome.

Earlier it was mentioned that patients often come up with very sound short term solutions to solve immediate problems and that those solutions are about taking the path of least resistance, substituting for what is not working right by exclusively using what is. The problem again, is that those solutions are very limiting. They eliminate adaptability and flexibility. Rather than just being able to "get up and go" or do more than one thing at a time, the patient moves in such a way that there is a discrete beginning and end to one behavior before he can begin the next. Recognition that a movement strategy enables the patient to do something that otherwise he is unable to do could be a powerful mechanism for motivating the patient to make the investment.

For example, one strategy for coming to stand in which the patient has some ability to proceed right into stepping, hold a cup, or stop part way is compared to perhaps the patient's chosen strategy in which none of those things are possible. The compensatory strategy obligates the patient to come fully upright, and he is unable to do anything else until achieving the end alignment and perhaps even getting the involved foot onto the floor. In comparing the two outcomes, the patient can readily identify the benefits of practicing what initially might be a more difficult or even a seemingly less stable method. When a patient asks the nurse on the ward—who is assisting him in a transfer from his wheelchair to the bed—whether he should do a "therapy transfer, or just the way he would do it," clearly he has not experienced the benefit of the alternative. Rather than viewing this as uncooperative, unmotivated behavior or related to cognitive or memory deficits, perhaps it is unreasonable to expect the patient would practice doing the transfer in a more difficult way. Why should he make the initial investment if he hasn't experienced what it buys him?

FORCED-USE PARADIGM/PROGRESSION

Recent clinical studies have demonstrated that by employing forced-use intervention, specifically restraint of the uninvolved upper extremity[10] combined with practice of functional tasks with the involved upper extremity,[5] the learned nonuse syndrome can be reversed. Commonly, the faster recovery rate often seen in the hemiplegic lower extremity as compared to the upper extremity is accounted for by the fact that both lower extremities are required to transfer and walk.[16] In other words, forced use occurs naturally as a consequence of the activities the lower extremity is engaged in. However, many of the gait deviations of hemiplegic subjects can be viewed from the perspective of overuse of the uninvolved lower extremity, with concomitant nonuse of the involved lower extremity. In fact, it is the opinion of the authors that the unilaterally involved patient develops a strategy for ambulation on level surfaces in which little if any support through the involved lower extremity is necessary.

Rather than meet the demands of loading response and single limb support with activation of hip musculature,[17] patients can be seen to "place" their involved limb and essentially push from back to front and hop over it with their uninvolved limb. In effect, this then is simply a variation of single-limb support, ambulation, as when an orthopedic patient with a fracture or ligamentous injury walks with crutches. Presumably because little if any force has been generated in the involved limb to counter the force of the push, the brief moment during which the uninvolved limb is unweighted is accompanied by what is essentially a "giving way" in the involved limb. Specifically, what is seen is a rotation back and lateral displacement of the pelvis, both of which serve to drive the tibia back and supinate the foot. The short, quick step or push from back to front with the uninvolved lower extremity is often followed by the tibia of *this* limb moving back and the pelvis displacing laterally, both of which hinder forward progression and create a pelvic obliquity whereby the involved limb is now relatively longer than the uninvolved limb.

Why would a person utilize a strategy which limits forward progression over the *sound* limb? The explanation may be that, again, this is a strategy for nonuse of the involved side in that rapid loading and acceptance of body weight is avoided. The problem is that because of the stance alignment of both limbs and lack of forward progression over both limbs, the task of advancing the involved limb is monumental. The mechanically advantageous alignment of preswing, which normally affords ease in clearing the foot, is lacking. Instead, the patient must resort to "lifting" the limb. The combination of elevating an already rotated back pelvis predisposes the limb to assume a classic abnormal extensor synergy complete with supination of the foot.

The appearance of this pattern has traditionally been attributed to the lesion and has therefore been seen as not readily amenable to physical therapy intervention. The above argument recognizes the biomechanical predisposition for this pattern, which can be said to result from nonuse of the involved lower extremity in the role of either accepting or supporting body weight. Verification for the biomechanical contributions to this pattern is found in observing that normal subjects assume an "extensor pattern," with alterations of tension in certain muscle groups when their movements are constrained to elevation and backward rotation of the pelvis prior to advancing a limb.

Based on the above discussion, one could argue that the patient would be capable of attaining a more ideal pattern for swing if the stance deviations of the two limbs could be resolved. Specifically, this would involve the patient's ability and willingness to challenge stance stability by unweighting and fully swinging through with the uninvolved lower extremity. This would help to create step length, whereby the involved limb could more readily attain a preswing alignment. Forward progression over the uninvolved limb would further enhance the ease with which the involved limb could swing, but it might then create a situation in which this limb was forced to accept body weight rapidly during loading response.

Clinical experience demonstrates that the patient often has the ability to accept and support body weight but that the natural tendency to compensate essentially eliminates the need to do so. Thus, in order to promote continual strengthening of the limb as well as to retrain a better swing pattern, therapy should be aimed at "forcing" the limb to participate in the support of body weight. Because this is a primary role of the lower extremities as opposed to fine manipulation of objects, forced use of the involved lower extremity could presumably be implemented earlier in a patient's rehabilitation program than forced use of the upper extremity. Ironically, though, it may be harder to implement, considering that restraint of the sound lower limb is unimaginable as well as unreasonable. In the following discussion, guidelines regarding implementation and progression of a forced-use program for the lower extremity will be presented (see Barton and Wolf[16] regarding guidelines for implementing an upper extremity forced-use program.)

Progression has traditionally involved sequencing the strength demands of muscles from less to more, or sequencing tasks from easier to harder. In a forced-use progression, however, the therapist should perhaps sequence tasks in a way that the treatment session proceeds from making it first *harder* and then *easier* for the patient to compensate. This may seen counterintuitive, and yet it is necessary, given the fact that the patient will automatically compensate unless the situation demands otherwise and that the demand may have to be great enough to get a response in the involved lower limb more automatically.

In a forced-use paradigm, progression can be viewed as the scaling of a number of parameters. One of these parameters might be a gradual removal of the body segments that make up the base of support, so that the involved lower extremity gradually takes over full support of the body. An electric mat table can be used to implement this approach in that as the surface goes up and the pelvis becomes less a part of the base, the feet constitute the greater part of the base of support. Then an additional demand on the involved lower extremity as part of the base is made when the patient now steps up on a stool, as can be seen in Figure 3-2. One should recognize that although the points of the base parameter may have been scaled up in terms of demand on the involved lower extremity for weight support, raising the mat table has created a situation in which coming to stand from this height has been made relatively easier. In this case, the parameter having to do with the *range* that that limb has to control through has been scaled down.

A second parameter that can be scaled is length of time for which the involved limb supports body weight. In Figure 3-3, the patient is now stepping onto a higher stool with the sound lower extremity, thus creating a situation that demands weight support on the involved limb for a longer time. Figure 3-4 demonstrates how a second parameter can be superimposed on the first. Having demonstrated the ability to support body weight on the involved lower extremity through longer duration, the therapist now takes away an additional

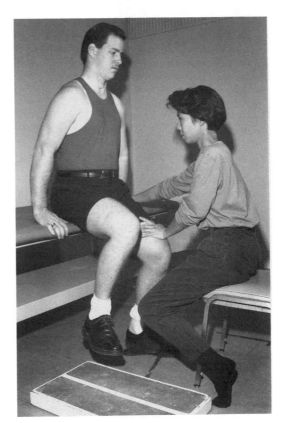

Fig. 3-2. Forced-use progression. Support through the left lower extremity is increased as the patient steps up on a platform with the right lower extremity.

part of the base by having the patient place his uninvolved hand on her head. The patient still has a point of contact with the uninvolved hand but perceives this contact as one that he cannot support heavily through.

A third parameter that can be scaled to promote use of the involved lower limb (while progressively increasing the demands on that limb) involves creating a situation in which the patient must link two behaviors together. In Figure 3-5, the patient has been instructed to stand up and take a step immediately with the right leg. In Figure 3-6, the patient is coming up to standing while holding a cup of hot coffee, which he hopes *not* to spill. Finally, in Figure 3-7, the patient is instructed to go off the surface toward his right side. Not only does this set up demand that the task be accomplished almost solely with his involved lower limb, but it is also promoting variety in the practice of this task.

Independence in moving from sitting to standing necessitates the ability to perform this task in a setting with changing environmental demands, such as a university. In addition to what has already been mentioned, progression can take the form of gradually challenging attentional demands by having the patient respond to a question while performing the task. As mentioned above, it is important to keep in mind that as one parameter is scaled up in difficulty, another might be scaled down. So, for example, in the course of the session,

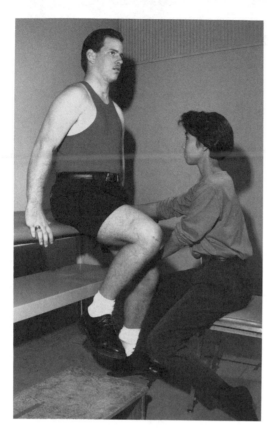

Fig. 3-3. Forced-use progression. Duration of support through the left lower extremity is increased as the patient steps onto a higher surface with the right lower extremity.

the patient may be able to come up to stand from the mat table in the lowest position utilizing both lower extremities equally. Now that the challenge becomes solely using the involved lower extremity to make that transition, as in Figure 3-7, it may be necessary to raise the mat higher and thus scale down the range parameter.

A critical progression that must be made to assure that the patient actually learns a motor skill (rather than just improving his performance) is the gradual withdrawal of verbal and manual feedback from the therapist. In Figures 3-2 to 3-4 the therapist is mostly providing boundaries and assuring that both the left upper and lower limbs of the patient maintain an optimal alignment from which force can be generated. Thus the therapist's right hand on the patient's left hand is controlling the option of the arm moving forward as the limb begins to generate extension force. This might help to assure that the force is being used to push into the surface as the patient unweights his uninvolved lower extremity. With her left hand, the therapist is putting slight pressure into the patient's foot to again give information about directing the force generated in his leg down into the floor. The therapist's leg is involved in providing a boundary for knee flexion so that the patient maintains an optimal alignment for

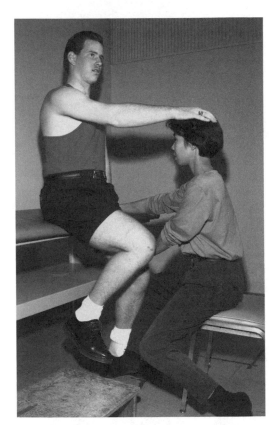

Fig. 3-4. Forced-use progression. An additional piece of the base of support is removed (right upper extremity) as the patient steps onto a high stool, thereby further increasing support demands on the left lower extremity.

pushing down into the floor. As the patient develops strength and control, the therapist must widen the boundaries by easing up on her manual contacts so the patient is forced to control through more range. The therapist is helping to provide an advantageous alignment for force production in weakened extremities, but the *patient* must solve the problem of keeping his trunk from pitching forward as he steps up with his sound leg, as in Figures 3-2 to 3-4, and standing off to the right, as in Figure 3-7.

A critical distinction between training and skill acquisition, made by James Gordon, clarifies the necessary role of the therapist.[15] He says that in *training,* the therapist gives the patient a specific solution to the motor problem; whereas in *skill acquisition,* the patient learns how to *solve* the motor problem. Rather than through verbal or manual guidance, in which the therapist takes the patient through each component part of coming to stand, the patient in Figure 3-7 must solve the problem of getting off the surface and going off to the right. Solution of the problem necessitates pushing with the involved lower extremity exclusively and thereby forces its use. In this example, the patient kept falling back to the left and thus was unable to accomplish the task. In successive attempts, the patient recognized that he was in fact "pushing" himself backward with

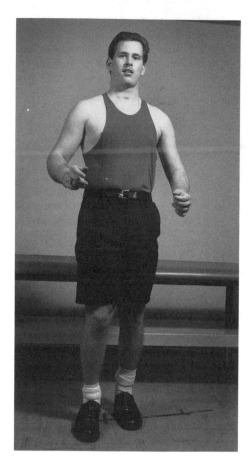

Fig. 3-5. Forced-use progression. Support through the left lower extremity is increased by asking the patient to stand and step as *one* movement.

his strong right leg. He was then able to solve the motor problem and come up to stand solely by pushing with the left leg once he stopped countering that force with the right leg.

In the examples of Figures 3-2, 3-3, and 3-4, it is possible to promote the patient's solution of the motor problem in a variety of ways. Rather than stepping up on the stool, the therapist can use an object the patient perceives as fragile. The problem becomes how to step onto an object with the strong right leg and not break it. The solution of this problem necessitates supporting the body weight through the involved lower extremity. If the patient fails to activate the involved lower extremity, it might lead to the breaking of a fragile object or in the patient's slamming his foot down hard on the stool. In both cases, the "error" is readily identified by the patient. In successive attempts, the patient begins to recognize that it is easy to move the strong leg if he holds with the involved leg. One outcome is compared to a different outcome, and what is driving the patient's performance is his wish to obtain the desired outcome, *not* the therapist's verbal instruction.

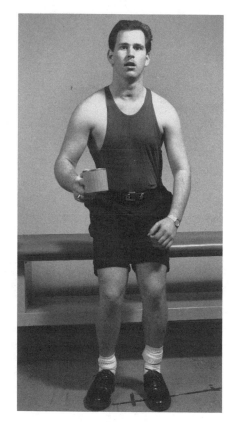

Fig. 3-6. Forced-use progression. Increased support through the left lower extremity is assured by the patient's ability to use the right upper extremity to push off the surface and by his interest in *not* spilling the coffee.

Preparation

In preparing to engage in a task, whether it is washing a car or playing tennis, an individual makes sure to have the appropriate equipment and sees to it that the equipment is in good working order. For healthy individuals as well as brain-injured patients, one's own body can be considered part of the "equipment" needed to perform functional tasks. One aspect related to whether or not *this* equipment is in good working order is if the mobility that is necessary for the task is present. So, for example, coming to stand requires extension of the lumbar spine, anterior rotation of the pelvis, and hip flexion to accomplish a weight shift forward and establish the feet as part of the base of support. Additional mobility at the hip, knee, and ankle is required to fully transfer weight to the feet and unweight the pelvis for ease in lifting off the surface. Although the majority of the weight transfer seems to be accomplished by moving into progressively greater ranges of hip flexion, there are mobility requirements specific for this task throughout the body. The scapula, for example, may seem remote from the action but could impede the ability to transfer weight forward if depression and adduction mobility is lacking. For the purpose of

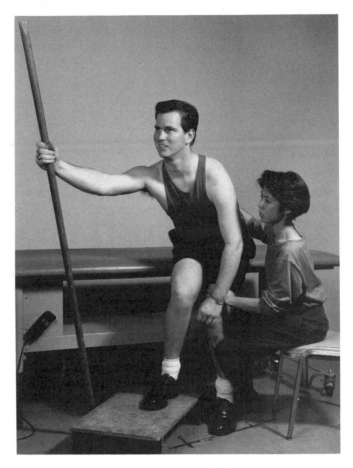

Fig. 3-7. Forced-use progression. By coming off the surface to the right, the patient has to push through and support almost exclusively with the left lower extremity.

this discussion, gaining mobility will be considered as one important aspect of preparation.

Range-of-motion activities have traditionally entailed passive movement of a limb, commonly with the patient lying in bed or on a mat table. However, there are tremendous benefits to gaining range with the patient in a more upright posture, such as sitting or standing. Probably the most obvious benefit of gaining range in a posture of function is that upon gaining access to mobility, the patient can immediately utilize it in a functional task. The therapist in Figures 3-8 and 3-9 is attempting to gain access to lumbar extension and anterior pelvic rotation range.[18] However, as the pelvis moves in relation to the lumbar spine, it also moves in relation to the femur at the hip joint. Moving down the kinematic chain, the femur potentially could move forward in relation to the tibia. In turn, the tibia moves forward on the talus. Proximal to the pelvis, there is the possibility that, as the lumbar spine extends, the thoracic and cervical spine

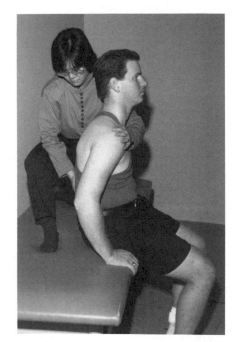

Fig. 3-8. Lower trunk stretching to achieve increased mobility toward lumbar extension and hip flexion.

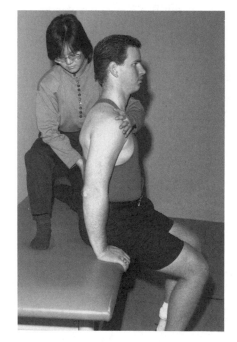

Fig. 3-9. By gaining mobility into lumbar extension and hip flexion, the patient achieves an anterior weight shift.

extend with a consequent adjustment of the scapula on a more extended thorax. Thus application of one technique has the potential to affect multiple segments such that a pattern of mobility is gained. Specifically the pattern of mobility that could result from this technique is lumbar extension; anterior pelvic rotation; hip, knee, and ankle flexion; thoracic extension; and scapular depression and adduction. Thus the patient is *prepared* to engage in numerous activities that utilize this pattern of mobility, such as lifting off the surface to pick up something on the floor, come to stand, or scoot back into a chair.

Traditionally, mobility of the limbs is gained as the limb is moved on a stable body. The technique depicted in Figures 3-8 and 3-9 is one whereby mobility is gained at the hips as the body moves on the limb. Gaining access to range by employing body-on-limb techniques has three very important benefits. One is that the movement that occurs replicates the task requirements more than when the therapist takes hold of the limb and moves it on the body. One may well move into 110° of hip flexion in order to come to stand, but it is not by the femur moving up on the pelvis. Second, when a therapist has hold of a limb with limited range, the patient may feel that he has little control in determining how far or how fast that limb is going to move. To guard against the limb being moved into painful range, the patient may actively resist the movement. Patients who are actively involved in moving their bodies on their limbs—whether it is sitting up straight and bending forward to move into increased hip flexion or rotating their bodies in relation to the humerus to gain range into external rotation—will report feeling more "in charge" and commonly push the limits into a painful range more than when they are passively moved by the therapist.

A third benefit relates to the pattern-of-mobility issue described above and is exemplified best by a clinical example. Prior to heterotopic ossification resection at the hip joint, a brain-injured patient had 30° of hip flexion range. The resection of the bone increased the range to 110° of flexion and postoperative physical therapy included "hip flexion range of motion." Over the 2-year period since discharge from rehabilitation and before resection, the patient ambulated independently in the community but was forced to sit with trunk flexion and pelvic posterior tilt to compensate for limited hip flexion range. Because of the inability to shift weight forward by flexing at the hips, the patient's only option for coming up to stand was to rock back and forth in order to generate enough momentum to lift off the surface. The surgical intervention may have increased the flexion range at the hip but it did not amount to a functional gain by altering the strategy for coming to stand. The patient was still forced to use the presurgery pattern secondary to a concomitant loss of lumbar extension and anterior pelvic tilt mobility. Utilizing the technique demonstrated in Figures 3-8 and 3-9, the therapist helped the patient regain low back extension and hip flexion range within a task-specific context.

The therapist in Figure 3-8 begins by increasing the tension in her hand, positioned above the ilium in the low back. This application of tension combined with the verbal instruction to "sit up tall" brings up an additional benefit of the technique. Even patients at presumably low cognitive levels will begin to move actively. The patient then is utilizing his own muscle force to move through the restriction and is thus resolving his own mobility problems actively through movement. In addition, the muscles that are being recruited are the very muscles that will be utilized to maintain the range that is gained. Therefore the possibility exists that muscle or movement reeducation and strengthening are occurring simultaneously with gaining mobility.

Clinical Hypotheses

Clinical experience has given rise to two clinical hypotheses[19]: (1) "Primitive" movement patterns can be modified by first identifying both the control and consequent components. Once the control component(s) is identified, it can be used to modify the movement pattern. (Historically, therapy has been directed at the consequent components, e.g., supination of the foot). (2) When voluntary control is limited or absent, practice with more automatic movements can be an effective means to initiate the retraining of voluntary movements.

The advantage of developing hypotheses is that they make predictions about outcomes that can be tested in an objective way. Generally this is thought of in terms of a large-scale clinical research project, but the fact of the matter is that every time a therapist makes a decision regarding intervention, it is based on some hypothesis he or she has about what constitutes the problem. The following discussion will assist therapists in making cause-and-effect associations between two (or more) observations and thus help in focusing treatment on the *cause* of movement abnormality.

The first hypothesis recognizes the biomechanical contributions to the abnormal patterns of movement observed in patients with a brain injury.

Historically, when a patient lacked selective movement and was observed to move in mass patterns of flexion or extension of the limbs, it was considered that the patient was in a "stage" of recovery in which there were no other options for movement. In fact, the patient might even be described as being "dominated" by a flexor or extensor pattern. Then therapy would be directed at controlling or minimizing the problematic component of the pattern.

For example, supination of the foot as a component of the extensor pattern creates an unstable base of support and could eventuate in a fall if a patient loads his weight on the lateral border of his foot. To avoid this problem, bracing, casting, tone-inhibiting techniques, and even surgical intervention would be utilized in an attempt to eliminate the foot supination. However, in analysis of total body movement patterns as patients attempt to perform tasks, it is very often possible to recognize that the appearance of the abnormal pattern is a probable, even predictable component of the total strategy. The emergence of the pattern in the limb can be linked to other component parts of the strategy, so that the question becomes: Is this a control component or a consequent component? The following clinical examples will lend support for the idea that these abnormal patterns of movement can be viewed as consequent components.

The outcome a patient might have when asked to bring his foot back by flexing his knee in sitting might be the *opposite* pattern of movement: mass extensor pattern of the lower extremity. As stated above, the therapist observing this outcome might describe the patient as lacking selective knee flexion, dominated by an extensor pattern in the leg, and that other options of movement are simply not possible. Analysis of the total body movement that occurs with the request to bring the foot back enables the therapist to recognize that the strategy used by the patient in attempting to perform the movement may predispose the limb to respond with extension. Perhaps the patient initiates movement and attains an alignment which "tips the scales" toward promoting extension and eliminates all other options. Commonly what occurs is that the patient leans back with the trunk, presumably to unweight the hip enough to free the foot from the floor. The initiation of movement in this way and the end alignment of hip extension may bias the system toward extension.

Support then for the idea that the extensor pattern is a consequent component of the strategy the patient utilizes to unweight the hip comes from the observation that when the therapist disallows hip extension as an option by physically maintaining the shoulders over the hips, the patient is able to flex the knee. The therapist may initially have to take some of the weight of the lower limb to optimize the ability of perhaps weakened hip flexors to slightly lift the femur. Eventually, with practice, these muscles are strengthened in a manner specific for the task. Much as in a progressive resistive exercise program (PRE), the therapist gradually reduces the support so that the patient ultimately accepts the full weight of the limb.

In the above example related to gait, the same argument can be used as that discussed in the section on forced-use paradigm/progression. The focus of the rehabilitation team might be the problematic components of the extensor pattern seen in the swing phase of gait. A brace might be used in an attempt to control the supination of the foot. Surgery or nerve blocks might be considered to selectively weaken or change the line of pull of overactive knee extensor, ankle plantar flexor, and invertor muscles. The problem here is that perhaps the effort is directed at the consequent component. In analysis of swing and stance deviations of both limbs as well as the interlimb dynamics, it is possible to conclude that the appearance of the extensor pattern is a *consequence* of having no other or better choice than pelvic elevation as the means to advance the limb.

The strategy of the patient to push from back to front with the uninvolved limb is presumably used to eliminate the need to support with the involved lower extremity. Additionally, in restricting forward progression over the uninvolved lower extremity by moving the tibia back, rapid weight acceptance on the involved limb can be avoided. These compensations of the uninvolved limb combine to eliminate a normal preswing alignment of the involved limb. Now, from a mechanically disadvantageous position, the most reasonable strategy for the patient to employ in order to clear the foot is to lift the leg by elevating the pelvis. The pelvis is often already in a rotated back position, and the combination of elevation and rotation back predisposes the limb to assume an extensor pattern.

As seen in Figure 3-10, if a patient is prompted to progress *forward* over both limbs as well as discouraged from elevating the pelvis if necessary, he demonstrates a more normal pattern for swing with hip, knee, and ankle flexion. In initial practice, a slider, which decreases the friction between the shoe and the floor can be used to promote the patient's ability to practice and strengthen the swing pattern with less concern of catching his toe.

It is not possible to conclude that the patient has *learned* a new strategy for swing until he can maintain the same level of performance without the assistance of the therapist.[20] However, the fact that he has the capability to execute a different movement option for swing when the control components of elevation and rotation back of the pelvis are eliminated lends support to the idea that perhaps therapy has been directed at the consequent components. To help patients actively resolve their problems (e.g., supination of the foot)

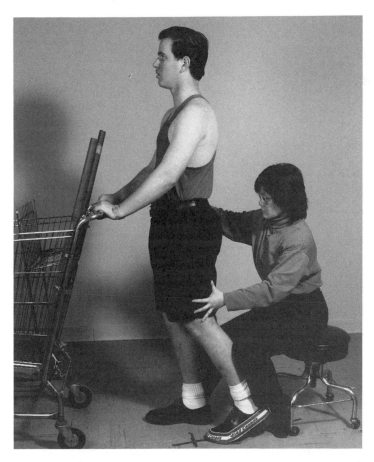

Fig. 3-10. Therapist discourages the control components of pelvic elevation and backward rotation on the left and thus enables the patient to utilize a more normal swing pattern.

through movement, it is necessary for the therapist to identify what is predisposing those problems to occur.

An additional clinical example serves to illustrate this first hypothesis but in addition leads to the introduction of a second clinical hypothesis. Commonly, when asked to move an arm, a patient with a brain injury will demonstrate a flexor pattern as the only option for movement. This observation can often be linked to the fact that this patient's strategy for arm lifting entails scapular elevation. This is a component that is not normally associated with the initiation of arm movement and presumably occurs in part due to weakness of shoulder musculature. Healthy individuals in an aerobics class can be observed to elevate *their* scapula after a number of repetitions of arm elevation. Remediating the problem of flexion as the only option of movement can be as simple as informing the patient *not* to elevate the scapula when attempting to move the arm. Eliminating this control component then, now enables the patient to demonstrate multiple options for movement of the arm.

In addition to informing the patient not to elevate the scapula in an attempt to lift the arm, the therapist may, at first, have to take some of the weight of the limb or shorten the lever arm by flexing the elbow, thus allowing the weakened shoulder muscles to perform optimally.

With his hand or forearm against a wall, a patient can practice and strengthen arm elevation by holding in increasingly greater ranges of shoulder flexion and abduction, depending on the orientation of the body to the wall. From here, the patient can attempt to control "letting go" of the shoulder eccentrically as the hand or forearm slides down the wall. This can be interspersed with attempts to push into the wall and hold at different ranges. If, however, by eliminating scapular elevation as the initial movement component, the patient is no longer able to move his arm or the situation is such that the patient was unable to move the arm voluntarily in the first place, then it is necessary for the therapist to consider an additional method for retraining voluntary movement.

This leads to the second clinical hypothesis, stated as follows: "When voluntary control is limited or absent, practice with more automatic movements can be an effective means to initiate the retraining of voluntary movements." This is related to the first hypothesis in that it requires total body analysis of movement in the performance of a task. One level of movement analysis is afforded to therapists as they observe movement and as they simulate the performance of a task. For example, in both scooting to the side, as one would do moving around a booth in a restaurant, and reaching for an object in sitting that is located high to one side, the arm that the body is moving away from serves to assist the shift of the body by extending or pushing into the support surface. Thus, these are two activities a patient could be involved in that not only have functional significance but could serve to automatically build extension through the arm into the patient's repertoire of movement options.

How precise in specification the lateral shift and reach need to be in order to promote extension through the arm may be related to the patient's initial capabilities. The limb is much less inclined to extend and push if the weight shift in sitting occurs from a flexed trunk posture or is initiated by the thorax moving laterally outside of the pelvis. So for a patient who has little if any ability to volitionally extend his arm, it may be necessary to specify the movement pattern more precisely. By initiating the weight shift from an erect trunk posture and with elevation of the side of the pelvis the body is moving away from, the scapula on that side depresses and adducts, which biases the limb even more to extend. The therapist may at first be involved in controlling the amount of initial elbow flexion, thereby optimizing the triceps' ability to generate force from a more ideal starting alignment. Patients may initially be unable to tolerate any deviations from the ideal starting alignment and movement pattern. In other words, the "window" of malalignment the patient can tolerate while still remaining able to generate a variety of movement patterns might be very small. By building those patterns in automatically, under more ideal conditions, it may be possible to strengthen the response and broaden that window.

TASK-SPECIFIC TRAINING

An important trend in rehabilitation is task-specific training. In addition to the fact that this concept is supported by research,[21-23] it seems logical that the more a patient can gain mobility, strengthen muscles, and practice movement patterns within a task-specific context, the more likely it is that there will be carryover into the performance of the task.

In reviewing the activities presented earlier, we can see that the gaining of mobility and the progression of weight support through the involved lower extremity were accomplished with the patient in a more upright posture. Progressively increasing the demands on one segment of the body can be looked at as a form of strengthening. But—as opposed to traditional forms of strengthening, such as leg lifts—it is one in which there is a specific organization of the whole body that is more like any number of tasks for an adult.

Only three areas of normal motor behavior have been extensively studied. These are gait,[24] responses to postural perturbations,[25] and the coordination of grasp and reach.[26] Beyond this, a therapist's understanding of a task is what is afforded him or her through observation and simulation of the task. There are a number of ways a therapist can use task analysis for treatment purposes. One way relates to the therapist's ability to identify deviations a patient might make from a more ideal strategy in performing a task. The level of analysis that is afforded a therapist through observation and/or simulation is one in which it is at least possible to identify movement components that seem to be a part of the task. In observing multiple performers, one recognizes that some of the movement components of the task are individual or variable while other components seem to be invariant features. Once the invariant characteristics are identified, a therapist can readily identify a missing or abnormal component in a patient's chosen strategy for task completion.

For example, there are probably several variations in how an individual might bring a cup to his or her mouth based on individual strength, mobility, experience, the shape and weight of the cup, and whether the person is upright or reclining. However, it is unlikely that a healthy individual would initiate that activity with scapular elevation, which is a component that is frequently seen as a patient with a brain injury attempts this task with an involved upper extremity.

Scapular elevation thus can be viewed as an invariant component, one that would never be present under normal conditions. As discussed earlier (see discussion of clinical hypotheses), scapular elevation might be a control compo nent that results in limited options for arm movement. Once the invariant components of a task are identified, they can be targeted in the treatment session. The following actual patient example illustrates the use of task analysis in identifying problems. The patient was a young man with a diagnosis of brain injury and demonstrating unilateral involvement.

The patient was interested in trying to regain skill in golfing but was unable to putt so that the ball would travel in a straight line. Instead, it would end up behind him and to his left. In analyzing the task of putting, one recognizes that the performer sets his posture, then turns his head to look at the hole, and then turns his head back to look at the ball. In observing this patient, it could be seen that this patient sequenced the task in exactly the same way. However, as the patient turned his head to the left to view the hole, the left scapula adducted and remained adducted even when he turned his head forward to look at the ball. Thus his alignment biased a left and backward trajectory of the ball. Therapy consisted then of gaining mobility in cervical rotation and engaging the patient in tasks that involved controlling the left shoulder forward while the head turned to the left, as well as practice in the actual task of putting. Once the patient had the ability to turn his head to the left but maintain the alignment of his body facing forward, he was able to hit the ball accurately.

The example of a golf putt lends itself to discussion of a second way in which task analysis can assist in treatment. Working on putting a golf ball may seem frivolous and not viewed as a priority for a patient who is limited functionally. Yet, it could involve several movement components that also apply to numerous functional tasks. A patient may be viewed as not willing to or cognitively incapable of participating in "weight shifting" activities, for example; yet when such a patient is involved in a task that he is motivated to perform and has experience with, such as playing golf, weight shifting occurs and is strengthened as a component of the task. The net effect is that a task is used to help the patient resolve his problems actively through movement.

SUMMARY

Currently, the scientific community is recognizing that the reorganizational capacity and the potential for recovery in the brain-injured adult is far greater than previously thought. In addition, the clinical community is beginning to identify that not all the behavioral deficits that result from a brain injury are lesion-driven but that some are more related to the propensity to compensate.

The strategies patients utilize for task completion are often good short-term solutions for solving immediate problems and accomplishing basic tasks, but they limit behavior and eliminate the need to recover strength and control of the involved body segments. In order to help the patient with a brain injury to recover and develop skills over a *lifetime,* the therapist must encourage the patient to learn to perform and recognize the benefits of alternative strategies that enhance functional capabilities.

REFERENCES

1. Mills VM, Quintana L: Electromyography results of exercise overflow in hemiplegic patients. Phys Ther 65:1041, 1985
2. Garland SJ, Hayes KC: Effect of brushing on electromyographic activity and ankle dorsiflexion in hemiplegic subjects with foot drop. Physiother Can 39:239, 1987
3. Kraft GH, Fitts SS, Hammond MC: Techniques to improve function of the arm and hand in chronic hemiplegia. Arch Phys Med Rehabil 73:220, 1992
4. Swaan D, van Wieringen PCW, Fokkema SD: Auditory electromyographic feedback therapy to inhibit undesired motor activity. Arch Phys Med Rehabil 55:251, 1974
5. Taub E, Miller NE, Novack TA, et al: Technique to improve chronic motor deficit after stroke. Arch Phys Med Rehabil 74:347, 1993
6. Connolly BH, Montgomery PC: Framework for assessment and treatment. p. 10. In Montgomery PC, Connolly BH (ed): Motor Control and Physical Therapy. 1st Ed. Chattanoga Group, Inc, Hixson, TN, 1991
7. Ogden R, Franz SI: On cerebral motor control: the recovery from experimentally produced hemiplegia. Psychobiology 1:33, 1917
8. Lashley KS: Studies of cerebral function in learning: V. The retention of motor habits after destruction of the so-called motor areas in primates. Arch Neurol Psychiatry 12:249, 1924
9. Taub E: Somatosensory deafferentation research with monkeys. p. 371. In Ince L (ed): Behavioral Psychology and Rehabilitation Medicine. Williams & Williams, Baltimore, 1980
10. Wolf SL, Lecraw DE, Barton LA, et al: Forced use of hemiplegic upper extremities to reverse the effect of learned nonuse among chronic stroke and head-injured patients. Exp Neurol 104:125, 1989
11. Ostendorf CG, Wolf SL: Effect of forced use of the upper extremity of a hemiplegic patient on changes in function. Phys Ther 61:1022, 1981
12. Henderson V: Predictive factors for functional recovery in adults. p. 9. In Rehabilitation of the Head Injured Child and Adult: Selected Problems. Rancho Los Amigos Hospital, Downey, CA, 1982
13. Kamm K, Thelan E, Jensen J: A dynamical systems approach to motor development. Phys Ther 70:763, 1990
14. LeVere TE: Recovery of function after brain damage: a theory of the behavioral deficit. Physiol Psych 8:297, 1980
15. Gordon J: Facilitation of skill acquisition in clinical settings. APTA Combined Sections Meeting. February 10, 1992; San Francisco, CA
16. Barton L, Wolf SL: Learned nonuse in the hemiplegic upper extremity. p. 79. In Gordon W (ed): Advances in Stroke Rehabilitation. 1st Ed. Andover Medical Publishers, Boston, 1993

17. Perry J: Gait Analysis. Normal and Pathologic Function. SLACK Incorporated, Thorofare, NJ, 1992
18. Bohman I, Utley J: NDT/Bobath 3 Week Course in the Treatment of Adult Hemiplegia, 1988
19. Winstein CJ: personal communication, 1992
20. Winstein CJ: Motor learning considerations in stroke. p. 109. In Duncan PW, Badke MB (eds): Stroke Rehabilitation the Recovery of Motor Control. Year Book Medical Publishers, Chicago, 1987
21. Winstein CJ, Gardner ER, McNeal DR, et al: Standing balance training: effects on balance and locomotion in hemiparetic adults. Arch Phys Med Rehabil 70:755, 1989
22. Richards CL, Malouin F, Wood-Dauphinee S, et al: Task-specific physical therapy for optimization of gait recovery in acute stroke patients. Arch Phys Med Rehabil 74:612, 1993
23. Malouin F, Potvin M, Prevost J, et al: Use of an intensive task-oriented gait training program in a series of patients with acute cerebrovascular accidents. Phys Ther 72:781, 1992
24. Patla A: Adaptability of Human Gait: Implications for the Control of Locomotion. North-Holland, New York, 1991
25. Frank JS: Earl M: Coordination of posture and movement. Phys Ther 70:855, 1990
26. Jeannerod M: The neural and behavioural organization of goal-directed movements. In Broadbent DE, McGaugh JL, Mackintosh NJ et al (eds): Oxford psychology series #15. Clarendon Press, Oxford, England, 1988

4 Management of Decreased ROM From Overactive Musculature or Heterotopic Ossification

DeAnna Anderson

Traumatic brain injury can have a devastating effect not only on cognitive function but on physical function as well. Joint contractures are a common complication following a traumatic brain injury. One study reports an 84 percent incidence of joint contractures related to an inpatient rehabilitation brain injury population.[1]

Joint contractures are secondary problems that develop from primary problems related to the brain injury. A person recovering from a cortical or brain stem lesion is often left with residual motor deficits, spasticity, tone, reemergence of primitive reflex patterns, and/or development of heterotopic ossification (HO).[2-6] These—alone or combined—can lead to abnormal posturing of an extremity, which results in the development of joint contractures if left untreated.

A joint contracture has been defined as a "chronic loss of passive range of motion (ROM) of a joint . . . because of structural changes in the nonbony tissues."[7] Physiologic changes in mammalian muscle fibers have been known to occur as early as 4 days after immobilization. Studies demonstrate that, relative to the limb posture, there are changes in muscle fiber length and in the number of sarcomeres in a series; in a shortened posture, there is an increase in the amount of connective tissue between muscle fibers. The *decrease* in the number of sarcomeres in series in a shortened posture is approximately twice the size of the *increase* in sarcomeres in a lengthened posture. Thus contracture formation occurs more readily than does the resolution of contractures.[7,8]

Along with the physiologic changes in the muscle fibers, there are physiologic changes in connective tissues to consider as well. Prolonged immobilization causes the proliferation of fibrofatty connective tissue in the joint space, and this connective tissue can eventually adhere to cartilage. Ligaments are composed primarily of collagen arranged in parallel fibers. The parallel fibers are oriented in such a way so as to restrict unwanted motion in a particular plane. Prolonged immobilization results in collagen fibers being laid down in a random order. This causes the ligaments to exhibit an increase in extensibility and a decrease in stiffness. Joint capsules are also composed primarily of collagen fibers. These fibers are woven in a criss-cross pattern, which allows for normal gliding between the connective tissue matrix. Prolonged immobilization of this matrix disrupts the normal criss-cross pattern and thus impedes capsular flexibility. Collectively, without an opposition force, the connective tissues are progressively shortened; this leads to reorganization of the fibers, thus increasing their density and limiting ROM.[9]

An imbalance in the activity of antagonist muscle groups acting across a joint is one of the contributing factors to the formation of joint contractures. In patients with upper motor neuron (UMN) lesions, this may be due to a combination of increased muscle activity or muscle weakness, or both. Prolonged contraction of a muscle can result in a fixed, abnormal posture and subsequent joint contracture. In the neurologic literature, there are at least six variant definitions of spasticity. Within the realm of this chapter, *spasticity* is defined as a velocity-dependent increase in a muscle's resistance to passive stretch.[10] It is seen as part of the UMN syndrome. Spasticity has two components, phasic and tonic. A phasic response is related to increased velocity of the stretch.[10,11] If the stretch is quick, clonus may be elicited. Another example would be a "clasp-knife response." A continuous resistance to passive stretch throughout the range produces the tonic response.

During an evaluation, the posture the patient assumes can affect the amount of resistance the therapist feels due to the labyrinthine influence. When evaluating spasticity, position the patient in an upright posture to elicit the maximal stretch response. When evaluating ROM, place the patient in a supine or side-lying position to decrease the labyrinthine influence, so that an accurate measurement of the joint can be obtained.[12] However, it is important to evaluate and compare ROM in functional postures as well, since it is in these postures that the patient will move and function throughout life.

The relationship between spasticity and abnormal movement is not clearly understood. Leahy[10] reported that Hughling Jackson categorized the dysfunction of neurologic impairment into positive and negative symptoms. Positive symptoms were described as spasticity or hyperactivity of the stretch reflex system. Negative symptoms were defined as deficits of normal behavior, such as the inability to move. Further, he concluded that these entities may be related but do not have a cause-and-effect relationship.[10] Studies by Sahrmann and Norton[11] indicated that motor deficits are produced by limited and prolonged recruitment of agonist contraction, by delayed cessation of the agonist contraction at the end of movement, and by overflow of contraction when movement is reversed. What does this all mean? It means that it is essential for a therapist to understand how movement occurs and how to interpret what is being presented. A therapist evaluating an *equinovarus contracture* may not realize that if a patient postures in hip elevation, this evokes an obligatory lower extremity extensor synergy pattern. When the pelvis is realigned to neutral, the lower extremity will relax and the foot will become more plantigrade. A therapist must analyze and interpret posture and its relationship to movement for an accurate evaluation. Therapists must focus on the ability to control movement as well as to manage overactive musculature.

In the event of joint contractures, accurate assessment of the major contributing factors is important. Cognition can be a major component in ROM loss. A person's cognitive function, related to attention and concentration, may be so severely impaired that it interferes with his or her ability to move the extremities.[2] In this situation, with patients exhibiting an LOC of I to III (on the Rancho los Amigos Levels of Cognitive Functioning Scale), conservative means of treatment can be implemented to maintain ROM. It is the physical therapist's responsibility to initiate and implement a maintenance program involving ROM to the joints, positioning the limbs in the bed and in the wheelchair, and instructing family members to perform these maneuvers throughout the day during the early phases of recovery. Prophylactically, the therapist can minimize the development of joint contractures by applying splints to maintain proper joint position until the patient's cognition improves. Ideally, the goal is to prevent the development of joint contractures. Prevention of contractures facilitates progression of the patient through the rehabilitation program, allowing the therapist to concentrate on improving function rather than managing joint contractures. Valuable time can be saved in overall rehabilitation if soft tissue contractures can be minimized or prevented.[2]

SERIAL CASTING

Unfortunately, many patients begin intensive rehabilitation with joint contractures already present, which then become the first priority of treatment. If passive ROM, positioning, stretching, and splinting techniques are inadequate to maintain joint position and mobility, serial casting or dynamic splints are the next treatment of choice. Serial casting has been used for over 20 years to manage and prevent soft tissue contractures in patients suffering from traumatic brain injury. "Serial casting can be effective and timely treatment for patients exhibiting decreased LOC who have begun to demonstrate soft tissue contractures or who have potentially deforming spasticity."[2] Casting provides slow, static stretch to contracted soft tissues and decreases the stretch response. Another benefit of casting is the total contact it provides to the extremity, which promotes relaxation of the muscle. Studies have shown that serial casting is most effective when administered within the first 6 months after injury, while the patient demonstrates ongoing neurologic recovery.[13] However, patients with long-standing and fixed contractures who are able to participate cognitively in a serial casting program may demonstrate some improvement in ROM.

There are several factors to be considered before initiating a serial casting program. The first and most important consideration is the patient's medical status. Some medical considerations include unhealed fracture sites, poor skin integrity, and accessibility of the limbs to monitor vital signs and to administer medications. These factors may require that the casting program be modified or postponed.

The extent of cognitive impairment is also a consideration. The patient may be agitated or restless, which could interfere with the ability to cooperate and relax for a successful cast application. Many times a cast may add to the patient's agitation and restlessness, and it can be potentially dangerous to the patient or caretakers if he flails his limbs as part of his agitation. In this instance, postponement of the serial casting program may be necessary until the patient has progressed through this stage or is chemically sedated.

Guidelines for Cast Application

The joints in the upper extremity most often in need of casting are the elbow, wrist, and fingers; in the lower extremity, they are the knee and ankle. Most casts are cylindrical in shape. The initial cast is referred to as the *resting cast*.[14] The joint is positioned in an easily obtainable range without being stretched, and is casted in this position. The therapist must be able to interpret the patient's response to the cast. The therapist should be able to determine the position in which the joint can be casted without undue pain or tearing of the tissues. The initial cast is left on for 7 to 10 days. The patient must be monitored closely for signs of swelling, pain, vasoconstriction, or pressure areas. After the resting cast is removed, a series of casts is applied at weekly intervals. Sufficient time must pass between casts to allow the cellular changes in length to occur. During cast changes, the therapist ranges the joint or performs joint mobilization to maintain or enhance mobility and assess motor control and skin integrity. It is important that the therapist pay attention to the arthrokinematics of the joint while performing ROM and joint mobilization so as to optimize increased ROM at the joint. Most serial casting protocols require a 3- to 6-week commitment from start to finish.[14]

Special attention must be paid when casting an extremity with increased tension. This increased tension can produce an increase in pressure against the cast and can thus lead to skin breakdown. For this reason, the patient's limb should be well padded, especially over bony prominences. Cotton as well as foam padding is used. However, it should be emphasized that proper joint positioning is crucial to minimize the potential for skin breakdown due to pressure. Once the padding is in place, the limb is wrapped in either plaster of Paris or fiberglass. The plaster cast requires 48 hours to dry completely. During this period, the patient should not bear weight on the extremity so as to maintain joint position and cast stability. A fiberglass cast, however, is able to tolerate full weight bearing 30 minutes after application without deformation of the cast. The disadvantage of fiberglass is that it is difficult to mold to the limb because of the speed with which it dries. Fiberglass is also more expensive than plaster of Paris. The therapist, therefore, must decide which material would be most beneficial and cost-effective for the patient. For example, for the more cognitively impaired patient (LOC I to III), plaster would be more appropriate because of the patient's inactivity. Patients whose programs include standing and gait training would benefit from a fiberglass cast, which lets them begin weight-bearing activities immediately after cast application. For the agitated patient, the fiberglass is more durable and can take more abuse. However, the restless patient may hurt or bruise other body parts with the fiberglass cast. Therefore, such patients must be monitored closely for their safety. Combination casts can be fabricated by wrapping fiberglass over plaster. This type of cast requires 24 hours to dry (Table 4-1).

Modifications can be made to the long cylinder cast to enhance its effectiveness and provide access to musculature, so as to incorporate other therapeutic modalities.[14] Dropout casts are modifications of long cylinder casts. Dropout casts are designed to allow aggressive ROM into extension but to provide flexion boundaries. For example, an elbow dropout cast is designed by cutting along the medial and lateral aspects of the posterior portion of the cast just

Table 4-1. Types of Casts and Their Indications

Type	Indication
Upper Extremity Casts	
Long arm cast	Applied when there is a loss of full elbow extension (30° or more). The long arm cast may or may not include the fingers and/or thumb (spica cast).
Short arm cast	Applied when there is a wrist flexion deformity. The short arm cast may include the fingers and/or thumb.
Finger and/or thumb cast	Applied when there are isolated boutonniere or swan neck deformities (or can be included in long arm cast or short arm cast).
Lower Extremity Casts	
Long leg cast	Applied when there is a loss of full knee extension; may or may not include the foot.
Short leg cast	Applied when there is an equinovarus deformity. The cast should extend distally past the toes to prevent the toes from clawing. Monitor subtalar position during casting to achieve optimal position.

distal to the olecranon process, leaving the posterior arm open. A knee dropout cast can be modified in two ways from a long leg (foot may be included) cylinder cast. One version calls for removing the anterior lower shell of the cast from the anterior to the medial and lateral femoral condyles to just above the patella. When the patient is prone, gravity assists the knee to extend unless the flexion contracture is more than 60 to 70°. If a patient has severe equinovarus, the lower half of the cast remains intact and the anterior thigh portion is removed from the back of the femoral condyles to just below the patella (Fig. 4-1). It is believed that this type of dropout cast is mechanically superior to the lower leg dropout because it maintains immobility of one of the two joints casted, providing more of a stretch across the knee. This type of dropout, as well as the elbow dropout, allows access to the extensor muscle groups, so that electric stimulation can be applied as a treatment option.[14]

The therapist must be aware of the potential for the limb to rotate within the dropout cast, also keeping in mind that once part of a cast is cut or removed, total contact is lost and the cast will expand slightly. Patients may use this "extra" room in the cast to put slack on the stretched muscle. This can lead to skin breakdown due to the amount of friction created between the extremity and the cast. This is a concern for patients who are cognitively impaired and restless. They cannot appreciate the importance of minimizing movement while in the cast; therefore, they are at risk for skin breakdown.

A knee dropout cast would not be indicated when the knee flexion contracture is greater than or equal to 60° because the effect of gravity as an assist is lost during proning due to the amount of knee flexion. An alternative to the dropout cast that allows access for other therapeutic modalities is a window

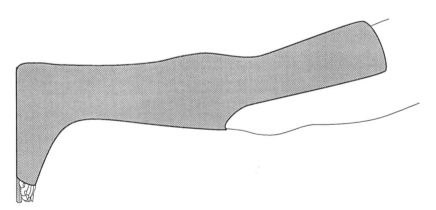

Fig. 4-1.   Long-leg dropout cast with anterior thigh portion removed. This allows access for other modalities. When the patient is prone, gravity assists the knee to extend unless the flexion contracture is more than 60 to 70°. If a patient has severe equinovarus, the lower half of the cast remains intact and the anterior thigh portion is removed from the back of the femoral condyles to just below the patella.

cutout, which allows application of electric stimulation. Contraindications for both dropout casts and window cutouts include the presence of edema in the limb.

Other modifications or additions can be applied to the casts for specific positioning purposes. Some common additions are spreader bars and outrigger devices. A spreader bar, used on bilateral lower extremity long leg casts, is placed between the legs proximal to the knees to prevent hip adduction. The outrigger is used in conjunction with a plaster heel cup and a bar that extends either medially or laterally to prevent internal/external rotation. These additions are most useful if they are removable for bed and wheelchair positioning. These additions may not be appropriate for confused patients; they may only increase their agitation and may even be harmful.

Wedging the cast at the knee is a convenient way of gaining range without removing and reapplying a new cast. The long leg cast is cut horizontally posterior to the knee and a piece of wood is then wedged into the space, forcing the cast into more extension. The cast is then replastered in this new position. This can be done to a cast only once. Care must be taken not to sublux the knee posteriorly when attempting to gain more extension during wedging.

Cast braces can also be used to maintain and gain ROM at the knee. The cast brace has hinge joints which align with the knee joint axis to allow flexion and extension. The joints can be locked in a specific position to allow movement in one direction and restrict movement in the other. Care must be taken to align the brace joint accurately with the knee joint axis so as to maximize function and preserve the arc of motion.

Another form of casting is referred to as *inhibitive casting*. Inhibitive casts are designed to inhibit persistent tonic reflexes.[8] Key trigger areas on the plantar surface of the foot are believed to reduce abnormal posturing of the foot. During fabrication of the cast, these trigger areas are used to aid in positioning a more desirable joint alignment. One may, for example, position the ankle in neutral or 5° of dorsiflexion, position toes in hyperextension, minimize pressure under the metatarsal heads, and apply deep pressure along the calcaneal tendon. This will help to relax the reflex and position the ankle in a more desirable weight-bearing posture.

Once the ROM goal has been achieved through casting, the limb is put in a final or holding cast.[14] This ensures the desired joint position and remains in place for 7 to 10 days. After the holding period, the cast is bivalved and converted into an anterior/posterior (A/P) splint. The amount of weakness around the joint, motor control unmasked, and increased tension remaining dictate wearing time of the A/P splint. In the case where a moderate increase in muscle tension may still be present, the patient may have to wear the A/P splint for 24 hours a day to maintain range. If a mild increase in muscle tension still remains, the patient may have to wear the A/P splint only at night. Treatment should entail weight-bearing activities that help to reduce the muscle tension in the involved musculature. Anterior/posterior splints are convenient in that they maintain the desired joint position but also allow removal of the cast so that the therapist may perform ROM exercises, reeducate and facilitate motor control, and carry out full-body bathing. Anterior/posterior splints are not appropriate for the agitated patients because their restlessness can pose problems. That is, as such patients thrash about in bed, they create friction within the splint. This can lead to skin breakdown.

Unfortunately, patients with impaired cognition have multiple issues besides joint contractures that must be addressed. Patients often have significant physical deficits, including muscle weakness and decreased motor control. Casting can be coordinated with other therapeutic efforts to promote and facilitate motor control and maximize function. A short leg cast can serve to break up extensor patterning of the lower extremity so as to allow proper wheelchair positioning and alignment (see Ch. 6). Both long and short leg casts can enhance a patient's posture and alignment in the upright position by stabilizing the joints distally. This allows the therapist to work on the trunk control and hip strength that are necessary for transfers and ambulation. As noted earlier, an upright posture can improve a patient's alertness and responsiveness to treatment. As the patient's cognition improves, so will his or her functional status. Clinical observations support the conclusion that weight bearing in lower extremity casts enhances the outcome of improved mobility as compared with non-weight-bearing activities.[2]

Misapplication of a cast can result in skin breakdown, with serious consequences.[2,8] The most common sites for skin breakdown are the olecranon process, the malleoli, and the calcaneus. Patients with low cognitive status are at high risk for skin breakdown due to their inability to communicate. For this reason it is imperative that the skin integrity be examined between each cast change and checked for discoloration of the fingers and toes. Inadequate padding or poor positioning of the joint contributes to skin breakdown. Look for imperfections or indentations within the cast—potential causes of skin breakdown—especially if the patient's program includes weight-bearing activities. Beware of late-onset neuropathy of the ulnar nerve and the peroneal nerve distribution caused by compression of these nerves. Wrapping the extremity too tightly may obstruct venous return and lead to edema. One way of checking this is if discoloration of fingers and toes lasts longer than 20 to 30 minutes. If this should happen, remove the cast. One last consideration is the need for special interdisciplinary team coordination to ensure that all priorities of the rehabilitative effort are addressed when casting multiple extremities.

DYNAMIC SPLINTS

An alternative to serial casting is the use of dynamic splints. Dynamic splinting proposes a functional system of low-load prolonged-duration stretching for resolving joint contractures.[8,15] The controversy over dynamic splinting versus serial casting is related to the viscoelasticity of connective tissue when stretched. When a stretching force is applied to the tissue and then removed, the tissue elicits both an elastic and a plastic response.[8] The elastic response is the recovery of the tissue to its original length, while the plastic response is characterized by permanent elongation. Optimal plastic deformation of the tissue occurs after prolonged periods of low-force stretch. The theory behind dynamic splinting is that remodeling of the tissue takes place and is triggered by the constant force being applied, resulting in a shift of the fiber cross links. By contrast, short periods of forceful stretching including plaster application in casting, result in actual tearing of the connective tissue.[8,15] This can result in additional collagen formation, thickening of the connective tissue, and often greater restriction in ROM, pain, and inflammation. Research demonstrates that short-duration, high-intensity stretch favors the elastic response, while prolonged-duration, low-intensity stretch favors the plastic response. Because of the viscoelastic properties of connective tissue, a low-load prolonged-duration stretch produces the greatest amount of permanent elongation with the least amount of trauma and weakening to the connective tissues.

Dynamic splints are designed with spring-loaded adjustable-tension devices. This allows the patient to wear the splint for a prolonged period of time while providing a continuous dynamic stress to the joint. There are several advantages to using dynamic splints.[8,15] One is that the apparatus can be put on and taken off by the therapist to range the extremity and to facilitate motor control through the newly acquired range and to enrich the synovial lining with blood supply. The only time to do this during a serial casting protocol is between cast changes. The second advantage is that skin integrity can be closely monitored, whereas with serial casting, skin can be checked only between cast changes. Additionally, one can increase or decrease the tension exerted by the device according to the patient's tolerance. This requires ongoing inspection of the skin for potential breakdown. There are several disadvantages to a dynamic splint. In the presence of severely increased tension in muscle groups, the patient is more prone to skin breakdown because the splints are not designed to have total contact so as to maintain even pressure (as do casts), which promotes relaxation of the muscle. Other disadvantages are as follows: (1) it becomes cumbersome to put on and take off the splint, (2) to splint over multiple joints within one extremity, (3) to align the splint joints with the anatomic joints to preserve the arc of motion, and (4) to preserve the effectiveness of the tension provided by the splints. Also, some patients may be cognitively or behaviorally noncompliant and may be able to take the splints off by themselves. Dynamic splints are more appropriate for patients with mild cognitive and behavioral deficits and with minimal to moderately increased muscle tension—as opposed to patients with pronounced cognitive and behavioral deficits and with moderately to severely increased muscle tension.

Progressive serial casting and dynamic splinting are two techniques that can be used in managing joint contractures that develop secondary to a traumatic brain injury. Their use in the early and acute stages is recommended, so that immobilization occurs while the patient's cognitive processes improve. The therapist must evaluate the most appropriate and beneficial technique for each individual patient.

ORTHOTIC MANAGEMENT

Once the desired joint posture has been reached, no underlying or only weak motor control has been unmasked or yet developed, or the increased muscle tension has not been relieved, then bracing and splinting are indicated. Orthoses and splints are designed to maintain the limb in a position that protects the spastic muscles from sudden postural changes; these may elicit the stretch reflex and aggravate spasticity.[12] The therapist may continue to reeducate and facilitate motor control while using orthoses and splints.

Orthotic management requires continual evaluation throughout neurologic recovery. Orthotic devices for the lower extremity are used to maintain ROM after a serial casting program, stabilize distally for gait training, protect tendons post-operatively, and provide support for the upper extremity.[12] Temporary orthoses are utilized in the early stages so that they can be modified as the patient's motor picture changes. Then a definitive custom-fitted device can be fabricated with more accuracy. Definitive bracing for lower extremities consists of a variety of ankle-foot orthoses (AFO). Definitive bracing to improve function in the upper extremity is rarely indicated.

If there is marked extensor weakness or increased tension throughout the hamstrings, a knee-ankle-foot orthoses (KAFO)—or a knee immobilizer with or without an AFO if the ankle joint is not involved—may be used during gait training until the muscle imbalance improves. The knee immobilizer is preferred over the KAFO because the KAFO is heavy and cumbersome to the patient. These devices are not designed for permanent use. They are difficult for the patient to don and doff and preclude the knee flexion necessary for the swing phase in gait. Frequently, the patient will not use such a device and will throw it away. If the increased hamstring muscle activity continues to interfere with knee extension, then surgery may be performed to eliminate the need for a KAFO or knee immobilizer.[12]

Usually an AFO is all that is necessary. AFOs are used to protect and stabilize the ankle in a desired functional position and/or to increase functional ability during gait. An AFO that restricts plantar flexion may be indicated to provide support during stance phase if a neutral ankle has been achieved through serial casting or by a posterior tibial nerve block. A rigid AFO not only stabilizes the ankle but also indirectly controls the tibia and stabilizes the knee by preventing ankle motion. Tibial control is important for the rhythm of gait, continual forward progression, and progression of the body over the foot. If a patient is unable to achieve a neutral ankle this causes a backward angulation of the tibia, impeding forward progression of the body over the foot. Consequently, the patient demonstrates a contralateral short step because he or she is unable to achieve a heel rise with a stable ankle and foot in the uninvolved stance limb. Conversely, the rigid AFO can stabilize the tibia if the patient tends to collapse into dorsiflexion, causing a forward angulation of the tibia.

Begin with a rigid AFO that has a double adjustable ankle joint (DAAJ), so the joint range can be adjusted as needed. The metal uprights should extend just distal to the fibular head, approximately 1 inch, to prevent compression of the peroneal nerve while allowing at least 100° of knee flexion.[12] A metal shank is fitted in the shoe to the length of the metatarsal heads to prevent undesired motion between the uprights and the sole of the shoe.

Once the patient has reached a stable motor picture or the postoperative swelling has resolved, a plastic polymer AFO can be fabricated. The plastic AFO can be rigid or flexible to allow motion at the ankle joint.[12] The thickness of the polypropylene and the extent to which it covers the ankle determines its degree of flexibility. Because of close skin and bone contact, proper fitting is crucial, along with frequent skin inspections for red areas.

Historically, lateral T straps were used with the idea of correcting a varus foot. They are no longer used except in rare instances. A T strap places excessive pressure over the lateral malleolus, which leads to skin breakdown. If the varus component cannot be controlled within the shoe or through motor reeducation, surgery may be performed to correct the position.

Orthotic devices for the upper extremity can be used to position the limb, aid in the prevention of joint contractures, and support the shoulder. An arm trough can be attached to the armrest of the wheelchair to position the shoulder and elbow in more normal alignment; the hand may be included as well. A wrist-hand orthosis (WHO) may be used to position the hand in neutral and prevent the recurrence of deformity after flexor tendon lengthening.[17] A wrist orthosis or splint should not extend to the fingers if finger spasticity is severe. For a subluxed shoulder, a sling may be used to reduce the subluxation.[17,18] It is important to remember that bracing or splinting is an adjunct to motor reeducation of the limb.

NERVE AND MOTOR POINT BLOCKS

A more aggressive, invasive approach may be necessary if a joint contracture is severe or if it is difficult to sufficiently maintain the range. This would include a nerve block or a motor point block.[3,13,17–23] A block is an injection of a chemical substance into the nerve or motor point that temporarily blocks the innervation of the muscles. Blocks are indicated when there is a moderate to severe increase in muscle tension that interferes with motor control and/or causes a decrease in ROM.[3,13,17–23] The chemical substances most frequently used to decrease spasticity are lidocaine or marcaine for short-term effect and phenol for a longer-lasting effect.

Local anesthetic nerve blocks are both therapeutic and diagnostic.[13,17] Therapeutically, nerves can be blocked prior to cast application. The anesthetic nerve blocks reduce spasticity by interfering with the gamma efferent motor fibers involved in the muscle stretch reflex.[13] This allows the muscles to relax, so that maximal joint correction and position can be attained prior to cast application. Diagnostic nerve blocks, using lidocaine or bupivacaine, are used to differentiate spasticity from myostatic contractures.[13] They also give a predictive preview for more permanent phenol nerve blocks or tendon lengthening procedures that may be under consideration. Lidocaine normally wears off in about 20 to 60 minutes, bupivacine in about 2 to 3 hours.

Phenol injection may be used when the spasticity is more severe and when there is potential for further spontaneous neurologic recovery. Definitive procedures such as neurectomies or tendon releases are not indicated at this time, since the patient's neurologic status may change.

The principal purpose of phenol injection is to interrupt the gamma efferent motor input temporarily so as to relax the agonist musculature, which can lead to joint contracture formation and interfere with limb function. This enables the patient to strengthen and gain control of the antagonist muscle while the agonist muscles are "put to sleep" temporarily and neurologic recovery is still occurring. Phenol injections may be performed by percutaneous injection of the muscle motor points, percutaneous injection to the peripheral nerve, or through open injection to the motor branches of the peripheral nerve.[17,22] Some functional potential should be present in the limb to maximize the effects of the phenol blocks.

Percutaneous motor point blocks are an effective tool in controlling mild to moderate spasticity. This procedure has the advantages of technical ease, bedside performance, and repetition as necessary. Motor point blocks do not produce complete relaxation of muscle tension, as do the peripheral nerve blocks. They do, however, allow more functional positioning as well as providing the opportunity for the antagonist musculature to be reeducated motorically. The most common sites for the performance of motor point blocks in the upper extremity include the pectoralis major, brachioradialis, wrist and finger flexor, and thumb adductor muscles. Motor points are located by nerve stimulators. The most contractile part of the muscle is the point of phenol injection. Enough phenol (5% aqueous solution) is injected at each site until minimal or no reaction can be elicited from the stimulator. After the procedure, the extremity is followed by progressive serial casting to correct residual deformity. Motor point phenol blocks can be repeated up to three times. The duration of the block is usually 1 to 2 months.[22]

Peripheral phenol nerve blocks may be preferred over the motor point blocks in patients with severe muscle tension. Direct percutaneous injection into the nerve provides complete paralysis of the muscle. The most important factor determining the amount of relief of tension is the accuracy of the phenol injection into the nerve.[13] A combination of motor point blocks and percutaneous phenol blocks may be indicated. For example, a patient presenting with moderate to severe increase in muscle activity in the elbow flexors may require both procedures. In this instance, a phenol motor point block of the brachioradialis muscle and a percutaneous phenol nerve block to the musculocutaneous nerve can be performed at the same time to reduce the tonic component of spasticity.[3] Some common lower extremity nerve blocks are performed to the adductor muscles and gastrocnemius and soleus muscles.

Open phenol nerve injections are selected over percutaneous injections if the nerve is mixed. Peripheral nerves commonly contain both sensory and motor fibers. An open phenol injection involves surgically exploring and identifying the motor branch of the mixed nerve. It is then injected with 3% phenol mixed with glycerine.[17,21,22] As in the case of percutaneous injections, a nerve stimulator is used to identify the motor branch of the nerve. Isolation of the motor branch will prevent loss of sensation and painful dysesthesia. Postoperatively, serial casting or dropout casts are used to gain and maintain ROM.[17,21,22] An open phenol injection is usually performed within the first 6 months of the neurologic recovery stage, when spasticity is most severe.[13] Its effects can last 3 to 6 months. It is hoped that normal or maximal neurologic recovery will be achieved by the time nerve regeneration occurs.

The most common sites for open phenol nerve injections are the musculocutaneous nerve and the posterior tibialis nerve. Indications for a musculocutaneous block are severe elbow flexion contracture resistant to serial casting and interference with hygiene of the elbow.[13,21] Indications for a posterior tibialis block are equinus contracture resistant to serial casting, excessive ankle clonus in weight bearing, and the inability to maintain the heel in the orthosis during ambulation (despite neutral ankle position at rest).[13,21] After an open phenol injection, the joint must be maintained by casting, splinting, or bracing.

According to Felsenthal,[24] phenol exerts two actions on the nerves. The first is a short-term effect, producing an immediate local anesthetic response which is directly proportional to the thickness of the nerve fibers. The second effect is long-term: the phenol causes coagulation of protein. Consequently, it is nonselective in the protein denaturation. This leads to Wallerian degeneration of the axons. The therapeutic effect of phenol therefore seems to be dose-related and nonspecific to fiber type destroyed.

The action of phenol and the Wallerian degeneration and regeneration accounts for the reversible tissue effects of phenol. This explains the return of increased muscle tension in some patients. There is a dynamic interaction between the effect of the phenol, the neurologic recovery, and the amount of aggressive therapy required to reeducate the antagonist muscle groups.[3,24]

SURGERY (NONFUNCTIONAL AND FUNCTIONAL)

Since spontaneous neurologic recovery can occur for a prolonged period of time, definitive surgeries are avoided during the first 18 months after the onset of the brain injury.[3,12,17,18,21] If definitive surgeries are performed too early during the recovery stages, permanent loss of strength or range can occur when functional neurologic recovery resumes.[3,21] If neurologic recovery is complete and the abnormally increased muscle tension reemerges 6 to 9 months following a nerve block, definitive surgical procedures would be indicated.

The team performs a full evaluation of the patient and the extremity to determine the need and goal of surgery. Some indications for surgeries include

(1) failure to maintain range through conservative measures due to overactive muscle activity, (2) to eliminate the need for an orthosis, (3) to gain functional improvement, or (4) for hygiene purposes. Definitive surgeries include neurectomies, tendon lengthenings or releases, and tendon transfers.[25] See Chapters 8 and 9.

Frequently multiple procedures on multiple limbs are indicated at the same time. The team must prioritize the patient's potential and functional status with care.

Interestingly, dynamic electromyographic studies have shown that pattern of muscle activity where tendons were transferred, lengthened, or released did not change after the surgery.[26,27] This demonstrates that excessive forces exerted by overactive muscles were reduced by the surgical procedure but the abnormal timing of the muscle activity remained the same. This reinforces the need for motor reeducation. Surgery can provide the necessary range for functional activity, but it is mandatory that the muscles be reeducated and strengthened in the newly acquired range for more efficient movement through therapy. Surgery is an additional therapeutic modality in rehabilitation.

BOTULINIM TOXIN

A new drug is beginning to emerge in the treatment of the brain injury population for controlling increased muscle tension. It is a purified protein, botulinim toxin, produced by the bacterium *Clostridium botulinum*. The toxin acts by paralyzing the muscle. It does this by rapidly binding to presynaptic cholinergic nerve terminals, preventing the release of acetylcholine and thus diminishing muscle contraction.[16,28–31] The dosage used is roughly proportional to the mass of the muscle being injected. The drug is injected right into the muscle belly. Side effects thus far reported are transient weakness, dysphagia for treatment with cervical dystonia, history of hypersensitivity to botulinum toxin, and infection at the site of injection. Also, since this drug has been used clinically, some patients have developed antibodies that block its favorable effects. These effects generally last for about 3 to 6 months. Repeated injections may be necessary. As with the other modalities, intense motor reeducation must ensue to promote maximal functional potential. The future role of botulinum toxin in the brain injury population remains to be seen, but it looks promising.

HETEROTOPIC OSSIFICATION

Another complication associated with brain injury is the formation of heterotopic ossification (HO), or abnormal bone growth around a joint. The etiology and pathogenesis of HO are unknown.[13,17,35] However, it is known that the formation of unwanted bone in a joint occurs in all planes following a brain injury and may be periarticular. Heterotopic ossification is commonly detected 2 months after the onset of the injury.[17,35] Clinically, the patient begins to feel pain and to lose ROM; the joint may be warm to touch.[17,35] Spasticity or muscle guarding is usually present around the joint. The alkaline phosphatase is elevated. Bone scans, which aid in the early diagnosis of HO, will demonstrate an increased uptake around the suspected joint. Radiographs confirm the HO diagnosis.[13,17,23,32,33,35] One thing to keep in mind is that a person healing from a fracture will also demonstrate elevated alkaline phosphatase. Bone scans can identify HO 2 to 3 weeks before the radiographs.

Once HO has been identified, the physical therapist should begin aggressive ROM and positioning to maintain range. Unfortunately, many patients cannot tolerate the ROM program due to the pain. This results in aggravating the spasticity and muscle guarding around the joint, making the ROM program more difficult to carry out. If the patient cannot tolerate the program and the heterotopic bone continues to grow, the joint may ankylose.

Prophylactically, the physician may prescribe diphosphonates to retard the calcification of collagen and osteoids. The diphosphonates may prevent the bone formation, but it does not appear to affect the process once it has begun.[13,17,35]

If the bone continues to grow, forceful joint manipulation can be performed under general anesthesia. The role of joint manipulation (i.e., its efficacy for ROM versus aggravating and enhancing the HO process) is still being studied.[34] In support of joint manipulation, it is performed as the heterotopic bone is growing to maintain range and to prevent ankylosis. Repeated manipulations may be performed if neurologic status improves. If it does not, joint ankylosis may be inevitable. Joint manipulation may be desired to place the affected joint in a more functional position for the patient when ankylosis is inevitable. Postmanipulation care includes ROM, use of a continuous passive motion (CPM) machine and 24-hour positioning regimens.

If the joint becomes ankylosed, the HO can be resected. Surgery should not be performed until the bone is mature, which will be approximately $1\frac{1}{2}$ years after the onset of the injury.[13,17,23,32,33,35] True bone cortex should be visible on the radiographs, the alkaline phosphatase should be normal, and the bone scan should demonstrate little or no uptake activity. If the bone is resected too early, there is a high recurrence rate, especially if spasticity remains around the joint. Once the bone is mature and resected, the patient is put on diphosphonates to prevent HO from recurring.[13,17,35]

The most common sites for HO are at the shoulder, elbow, hip, and knee, although it can occur at other joints.[13,17,23,32,33,35] Ankylosis of the elbow and hip are most common. When HO develops in the shoulder, significant shoulder disability is rare. The patient usually complains of decreased ROM and some pain. In the elbow, bone usually forms anteriorly or posteriorly. The site of heterotopic bone correlates with the posture of the extremity.[13] Anterior bone formation is more difficult to manage than posterior bone formation. By the time anterior bone matures, a flexion contracture has usually developed. During the early stages of bone maturation, a phenol nerve block to the musculocutaneous nerve can be performed to decrease spasticity about the joint in the hopes of maintaining a desirable ROM. Resection of the bone is difficult because of the neurovascular anatomy within the joint.

The hip has three heterotopic bone locations; anterior, medial, and posterior.[13,17,32,33,35] Anterior bone resection usually meets with excellent results for improving hip ROM. Medial bone resection also provides good results with ROM. Early percutaneous or open adductor myotomy and obturator neurectomy are useful in maintaining hip abduction. The posterior bone formation about the hip is the most serious. Hip flexion contractures are almost always present.[13] Resection of the bone may not always be helpful since the flexion contracture already exists. In this case, a proximal femur extension osteotomy is performed to obtain more range. In the knee, HO formation is rare but will sometimes occur. It can usually be managed by aggressive ROM, without surgery.

Positioning around the clock is important for maintaining ROM. Passive ROM and CPM should also be initiated 3 to 5 days postoperatively to keep the joint surfaces lubricated. For the lower extremity, when the patient is cleared by the surgeon for weight bearing, motor reeducation and strengthening in function should begin. Commonly, functional hip ROM is obtained after surgery. However, it is not uncommon for the patient to revert back to compensatory postures and movements after the bone has been resected. The patient does not know how to use the newly gained ROM. Motor reeducation and strengthening in function are therefore important, so that the patient can become more efficient with movement and function. A more creative and beneficial method to gain ROM can be seen when ranging the body on the limb versus the limb on the body. It is more meaningful and functional for the patient to have 110° of hip flexion in sitting and flexing forward to come to stand than it is for the patient to have 110° of hip flexion supine with passive ROM. The postoperative goal is to reeducate and strengthen the muscles in the newly acquired range *through function* so that the patient becomes more efficient with movement and the activities of daily living.

If the patient has good neurologic recovery or demonstrates some motor control about the joint, the results of surgery result in increased ROM. If spasticity remains about the joint, there is a high incidence of recurrence of HO formation and a significant gain in ROM is unlikely. The best single prerequisite for a good surgical result with the lowest recurrence rate of HO is a patient with minimal cognitive and minimal to moderate physical disability. These patients tend to demonstrate improved function of the limb and a low recurrence rate for new bone formation. In contrast, patients with moderate to severe cognitive deficits and severe physical deficits showed no improvement in function and had a high recurrence rate for new bone formation.[33]

Clinically, brain injury manifests itself differently in each person. The extent of motor loss, abnormal muscle tension, tone, primitive reflexes, HO formation, and cognitive deficit varies from patient to patient. Close interdisciplinary team efforts are essential to a well-organized and beneficial rehabilitation program. Prevention of joint contractures is the ultimate therapeutic team goal. Unfortunately, joint contractures are a common problem.

Conservative measures should be considered first in managing the contractures. Acutely, while the patient is still in a coma or at a low cognitive stage (LOC I to III), passive ROM, positioning, splinting, and family education should be emphasized in an attempt to prevent the development of joint contractures. If the patient has already developed joint contractures, serial casting or dynamic splinting should be initiated. The patient's cognitive status and the amount of increased tension in the extremity will aid in the decision process for determining the most appropriate approach to be taken. Treatment techniques focusing on motor control must be included along with the casting or splinting program. It is essential to reestablish active motor control. In assessing the patient, keep in mind that postural alignment and stability directly influence quality of movement and the amount of muscle overactivity in the extremities. In a casting program, variations in the cast may augment the use of other modalities.

If the team members believe they are unable to manage the joint contractures satisfactorily due to the increased muscle activity, nerve blocks can be performed. A motor point or nerve block may be used therapeutically or diagnostically to aid in the management program of the joint contracture. Temporary nerve blocks may be used in conjunction with a serial casting program to temporarily reduce muscle activity. If this method is not effective, phenol may be used, with longer-lasting results. An alternative to phenol nerve injections is the injection of botulinum toxin into the muscle. This drug is new to the brain injury population and its results are still being studied.

If no underlying motor control has been unmasked and the muscle overactivity continues to interfere with positioning and movement, more definitive surgery may be indicated (see Chs. 8 and 9). The surgeries may be of nonfunctional or of functional stature. Nonfunctional surgeries pertain to hygiene and positioning goals. Functional surgeries are performed to improve function of the extremity and allow it to become brace free. Such surgeries include neurectomies, tendon lengthenings, tendon releases, and tendon transfers. An important aspect of the decision-making process is the patient's cognitive status, his or her ability to participate in postoperative treatment, and the amount of motor control present. Surgeries are followed with emphasis on positioning, bracing, or splinting and motor reeducation to the extremity.

In regard to the management of HO, ROM and positioning should be initiated immediately once the heterotopic bone is suspected. Blocks may be performed to help control the spasticity around the joint. Joint manipulations are performed to maintain ROM and to prevent ankylosis. If neurologic recovery continues, repeated joint manipulations can be performed. Sometimes joint ankylosis is inevitable and surgical resection is indicated. Surgery should not be performed until the HO bone is mature, approximately 18 months after the onset of the injury. Alkaline phosphate levels should be normal, bone scans should show little or no uptake activity, and radiographs should show mature bone before surgery is undertaken.

Postoperative treatment, regardless of the type of surgical intervention, is emphasized. Once ROM has been regained, the patient must utilize that range to avoid losing it again. A patient with cognitive impairment benefits more from a program that is structured to strengthen and reeducate the muscles through function than through traditional unrelated strengthening and ROM exercises.

REFERENCES

1. MacKay-Lyons M: Low-load, prolonged stretch in treatment of elbow flexion contractures secondary to head trauma: a case study. Phys Ther 69:50, 1989
2. Zablotny C, Forte Andric M, Gowland C: Serial casting: clinical applications for the adult head-injured patient. J Head Trauma Rehabil 2:46, 1987
3. Keenan ME, Tomas ES, Stone L, Gersten LM: Percutaneous phenol block of the musculocutaneous nerve to control elbow flexor spasticity. J Hand Surg 15A:340, 1990
4. Keenan ME, Romanelli RR, Lunsford BR: The use of dynamic electromyography to evaluate motor control in the hands of adults who have spasticity caused by brain injury. J Bone Joint Surg 71A:120, 1989
5. Keenan ME, Thomas TH, Stone LR: Dynamic electromyography to assess elbow spasticity. J Hand Surg 15A:607, 1990
6. Keenan BE, Crieghton J, Garland DE, Moore T: Surgical correction of spastic equinovarus deformity in the adult head trauma patient. Foot Ankle 5:35, 1984
7. Lehmkuhl LD, Thoe LL, Baize C et al: Multimodality treatment of joint contractures in patients with severe brain injury: cost, effectiveness, and integration of therapies in the application of serial/inhibitive casts. J Head Trauma Rehabil 5: 23, 1990
8. Hepburn BR: Case studies: contracture and stiff joint management with Dynasplint. J Orthop Sports Phys Ther 498, 1987
9. Sapega AA, Quedenfeld TC, Mover RA, Butler RA: Biophysical factors in range of motion exercises. Phys Sportsmed 9:57, 1981
10. Leahy P: Motor control assessment. p. 69. In Montgomery P, Connolly B (eds): Motor Control and Physical Therapy Theoretical Framework and Practical Application. Chattanooga Group Inc. Hixson, NJ, 1991
11. Sahrmann SA, Norton BJ: The relationship of voluntary movement to spasticity in the upper motor neuron syndrome. Ann Neurol 2:460, 1977
12. Waters RL, Garland DE, Montgomery J: Orthotic prescription for stroke and head injury: specific applications. pp. 270–286. In Bunch WH: Atlas of Orthotics. 2nd Ed. CV Mosby, St Louis, 1985
13. Garland DE: Head injuries in adults. In Nickel VL (ed): Orthopedic Rehabilitation. Nickel (ed): Churchill Livingstone, New York, 1982
14. Booth BJ, Doyle M, Montogomery J: Serial casting for the management of spasticity in the head-injured adult. Phys Ther 63:1960, 1983
15. Hepburn GR: The Dynasplint system for resolution of immobilization stiffness and established contractures. Dynasplint Systems, Severna Park, MD, 1987
16. Jankovic J, Brin MF: Therapeutic uses of botulinum toxin. N Engl J Med 324:1186, 1991
17. Keenan ME: Management of the spastic upper extremity in the neurologically impaired adult. Clin Orthop Rel Res 223:116, 1988

18. Garland DE, Keenan ME: Orthopedic strategies in the management of the adult head-injured patient. Phys Ther 63:2004, 1983

19. Keenan ME, Botte MJ: Technique of percutaneous phenol block of the recurrent motor branch of the median nerve. J Hand Surg 12A:806, 1987

20. Keenan ME, Todderud EP, Henderson R, Botte M: Management of intrinsic spasticity in the hand with phenol injection or neurectomy of the motor branch of the ulnar nerve. J Hand Surg 12A:734, 1987

21. Garland DE, Lucie R, Waters RL: Current uses of open phenol nerve block for adult acquired spasticity. Clin Orthop Rel Research 165:217, 1982

22. Garland DE, Lilling M, Keenan ME: Percutaneous phenol blocks to motor points of spastic forearm muscles in head-injured adults. Arch Phys Med Rehabil 64:243, 1984

23. Garland DE, Rhoades ME: Orthopedic management of brain-injured adults. Clin Orthop Rel Res 131:111, 1978

24. Felsenthal G: Pharmacology of phenol in peripheral nerve blocks: a review. Arch Phys Med Rehabil 55:13, 1974

25. Keenan ME: Surgical decision making for residual limb deformities following traumatic brain injury. Orthop Rev 17:1185, 1988

26. Waters RL, Frazier J, Garland DE, et al: Electromyographic gait analysis before and after operative treatment for hemiplegic equinus and equinovarus deformity. J Bone Joint Surg 64:284, 1982

27. Keenan ME, Ure K, Smith CW, Jordan C: Hamstring release for knee flexion contracture in spastic adults. Clin Orthop 236:221, 1988

28. Kinash RG, Fulton NJ: Botulinum toxin for blepharospasm: challenges for rehabilitation nurses. Rehab Nurs 16:184, 1991.

29. Assessment: The Clinical Usefulness of Botulinum Toxin-A in Treating Neurological Disorders. Report of the Therapeutics and Technology Assessment Subcommittee of the American Academy of Neurology, 1990

30. Snow BJ, Tsui JKC, Bhatt MH, et al: Treatment of spasticity with botulinum toxin: a double-blind study. Ann Neurol 28:4, 1990

31. Das TK, Park DM: Effect of treatment with botulinum toxin on spasticity. Postgrad Med J 65:208, 1989

32. Garland DE, Blum CE, Waters RL: Periarticular heterotopic ossification in head-injured adults. J Bone Joint Surg 67A:1143, 1980

33. Garland DE, Hanscom DA, Keenan ME, et al: Resection of heterotopic ossification in the adult with head trauma. J Bone Joint Surg 67A:1261, 1985

34. Garland DE, Razza BE, Waters RL: Forceful joint manipulation in head-injured adults with heterotopic ossification. Clin Orthop 169:133, 1982

35. Marinissen JC: Management of heterotopic ossification following traumatic brain or spinal cord injury. Orthop Phys Ther Clin North Am 2:71, 1993

5 | Evaluation and Management of Swallowing Dysfunction

Cynthia M. Zablotny

Many of the social interactions in everyday life revolve around the all-important task of eating. It is not surprising, then, that experiencing impairment in the physiologic process of swallowing, as is frequently seen following traumatic brain injury, represents a significant functional loss for any patient. Conversely, the remediation of these swallowing deficits can serve as an important milestone in a patient's recovery process. This is especially true for the severely involved patient who may be otherwise incapable of performing even the most simple activity of daily living. Regaining the ability to swallow at least some foods safely can be instrumental in the restoration of some basic human dignity.

The management of swallowing dysfunction in the brain-injured patient involves the support and expertise of an interdisciplinary team. Although the primary swallowing therapist may vary from one facility to the next, the physical therapist should recognize the various skills and tools he or she can offer the patient with impairment in this process. Our understanding of kinesiology and of the neuroanatomic structures and neurophysiologic processes involved in swallowing is of great assistance in evaluating the patient with deglutition disorders. Furthermore, the physical therapist's background in the use of various facilitative techniques for muscle strengthening or reeducation can be used to develop a comprehensive treatment approach to address swallowing deficits and related problems with respiration and coughing.

99

INCIDENCE OF AND RECOVERY FROM SWALLOWING DYSFUNCTION FOLLOWING TRAUMATIC BRAIN INJURY

Only a few authors have actually detailed the incidence of swallowing problems in the traumatic brain injury population. Winstein performed a retrospective chart review of 201 brain-injured patients admitted to an inpatient rehabilitation program and revealed a 27 percent incidence of some type of swallowing disorder among these patients.[1] Of those with deglutition problems, 82 percent were incapable of oral feeding at the time of admission, while the remaining 18 percent were able to handle at least a pureed diet while still demonstrating associated swallowing difficulties. Winstein reported that the most frequently identified problem interfering with swallowing in the brain-injured population she studied was cognitive impairment, followed by the occurrence of deficits in motor control.

Further examination of the incidence of swallowing dysfunction in the brain-injured population was performed by Lazarus and Logemann in a study involving 53 patients.[2] These researchers categorized their findings into a set of nine separate swallowing motility problems that further delineated the exact motor control deficits seen in the brain-injured patient. Those deficits seen most frequently included problems with triggering a swallow, decreased tongue control, and decreased pharyngeal peristalsis.

More recently, Cherney and Halper reported data supporting the relationship between cognitive-communicative and behavioral deficits and the incidence of swallowing dysfunction in the brain-injured patient.[3] They noted that 61 percent of the patients they studied presented with severe oral intake deficits and concomitantly severe cognitive and communicative deficits. Conversely, only 6 percent of their patients with moderate or mild cognitive impairments also presented with severe oral intake problems.

Reports of success in improving oral intake ability during the rehabilitative process vary greatly.[1,3] Despite this variation, it is generally noted that the recovery of swallowing abilities occurs gradually and frequently parallels cognitive recovery. One author reported that the return of functional oral feeding occurred within 5 months from the time of onset in the majority of patients with traumatic brain injury in her study.[1]

These studies support the identification of swallowing dysfunction among patients with a traumatic brain injury as a significant clinical problem facing the rehabilitation team. Many factors influence the degree of impairment and prognosis for recovery of swallowing abilities. The rehabilitation team dealing with this problem is faced with the task of addressing all the components of this issue to most efficiently and effectively remediate the clinical deficits.

PATIENT EVALUATION

Many authors have detailed the phase-specific mechanics of the swallowing process.[4-6] An understanding of this information is implicit to the evaluation of swallowing dysfunction in any patient population. A knowledge of normal function allows for accurate comparisons when dysfunction is suspected. The information in this chapter assumes a basic understanding of these normal mechanics.

Initial assessment of the swallowing problems of a brain-injured patient begins with a thorough chart review. Pertinent facts to review include the type of brain trauma sustained, the lesion site, the patient's age, and time from onset of injury. These factors have predictive value with respect to the patient's overall potential for recovery.[2,7] It is also necessary to gain an understanding of the history of the patient's swallowing difficulties to date by looking for information documenting nutritional management since the time of onset, the length of intubation if appropriate, and the presence of aspiration pneumonia or other respiratory problems. Additionally, the therapist should be aware of any problems such as facial fractures which might affect the structures involved in the swallowing process.

Initial patient observation can provide the therapist with a great deal of information related to swallowing capabilities. It is ideal to perform a screening assessment in a quiet environment that is free of distractions. Observation of the patient will provide the therapist with information regarding the patient's abilities to attain and maintain adequate head and trunk alignment. Any abnormal postures of the head, neck, trunk, or upper extremities can be observed, as any of these may place the swallowing structures in a position of malalignment that makes swallowing less efficient and less safe. Asymmetries in motor control involving the face should be noted, as well as the patient's ability to handle secretions. Frequent drooling may indicate a sensory, motor, or cognitive deficit. If the patient is verbal, voice quality, breath control, and ability to articulate can also be assessed.

Physical Examination

Assessment of the physical structures involved in deglutition is best accomplished using a systematic approach that parallels the normal swallowing process. The success of this evaluation depends partly upon the patient's level of alertness and attentiveness to the tasks he or she is being asked to do. These factors will directly influence the amount of useful information the therapist might be able to gather in a single evaluation session. Realistically, the best evaluation results will be obtained if the patient is assessed over a period of several days and at various times of each day. In addition to assessing the patient's ability to attend to a specific task, it is important to evaluate memory capabilities and behavioral traits such as impulsivity and judgment, as problems with any of these may influence the management of the patient's overall swallowing program.

Assessment of Head, Neck, and Trunk Control

The purpose of a postural assessment is to determine whether the patient has adequate mobility and motor control for maintaining good head and neck alignment to optimize the efficiency of the swallowing structures. The normal individual can easily demonstrate the importance of this alignment by attempting to swallow some food with the head rotated, or laterally flexed to one side, or allowed to hang forward in a posture of extreme cervical and capital flexion, or with the head in a combined posture of cervical flexion with capital extension.[8] All of these postures make it more difficult for even the normal individual to swallow despite intact motor control capabilities. These postures might be seen in a brain-injured patient lacking adequate head and trunk control, and they serve to detract from such a patient's overall effectiveness in completing the swallowing process.

Both active and passive mobility of the head and neck are assessed to determine how easily a neutral midline posture can be attained and held. If the patient is capable of sitting up in a wheelchair or on the edge of the bed, the therapist will be able to determine the effect of the patient's preferred trunk posture on head and neck positioning. If appropriate, the therapist can ask the patient to realign himself to determine the effectiveness of his own postural corrections. The therapist may have to facilitate this process manually with some patients. The information gained through this assessment is useful in planning a treatment program involving manual facilitative techniques to improve postural control, prescribing appropriate wheelchair modifications, and determining whether the patient can best be positioned in bed or wheelchair for possible future feeding trials.

Orofacial Examination

Response to Cutaneous Stimulation

The first step in assessing the orofacial structures that are active in the oral phase of swallowing involves an evaluation of the patient's response to cutaneous input. This evaluation enables the therapist to detect the presence or absence of abnormal orofacial reflexes as well as any tendency toward oral defensiveness. The persistence of abnormal reflexes in a patient several months after onset is usually indicative of a more severe clinical picture.[9] Reflexes that should be examined include a rooting response, which is stimulated through the application of a light stroking input away from the corners of the mouth. The response of the patient may be to turn the head toward the stimulus, although the patient may also root away from the stimulus. The latter response is more apt to interfere with any future feeding attempts. The stimulus for a bite reflex is delivered through the application of digital pressure to the center of the lips against the teeth. The bite reflex is present if this stimulus promotes a repetitive up and down motion of the jaw. A tongue thrust may also be noticed following any type of tactile stimulation to the lips or perioral region. Light pressure to the center of the lips may instead elicit lip protrusion or a pursing response. The therapist may find that some of these responses directly interfere with further assessment of the oral cavity and with any attempts at feeding that otherwise might be indicated. Dealing with these reflexes can be a critical issue in helping the more severely involved patient to progress through the initial phases of a swallowing program.

Strength and Mobility of the Perioral Structures

Functional assessment of the facial muscles involved in swallowing can be performed if the patient is capable of following verbal commands or imitating postures. The goal of this assessment is to determine whether each specific assessed motion is functional enough to contribute to the overall mechanics of the swallowing process. For example, the patient's skill in maintaining lip closure is assessed by applying manual resistance to the patient's attempt to keep the lips closed. Functional lip closure implies that the patient has adequate strength to maintain this position without allowing any leakage of saliva. Weak functional control for this activity implies decreased strength when compared to normals, yet still the ability to prevent drooling. Nonfunctional lip closure implies that weakness prevents the maintenance of an adequate seal about the lips and allows for drooling. Other actions involving the face that are assessed using a similar grading system include the ability to pucker the lips, smile, close the lips around a straw, and compress the cheeks in against a tongue blade. Nonfunctional motor control involving one or more of these activities may contribute to drooling, pocketing of food in the cheeks, or an inability to keep food in the oral cavity while chewing.

It is essential that jaw opening and closing abilities be assessed to determine whether food may easily enter the mouth and be held therein. In the normal individual, jaw opening should be approximately 35 to 40 mm and lateral deviation should be approximately 10 mm.[10,11] It is not uncommon for a brain-injured patient whose medical history includes a prolonged length of coma or the presence of primitive responses such as a bite reflex to present with significant reductions in jaw opening capabilities. Jaw retraction is commonly seen in these patients as a result of prolonged supine positioning or abnormal facial muscle tonus.

Intraoral Responses and Sensation

Assessment of intraoral responses to cutaneous input helps the therapist determine the location and type of stimulus responsible for producing both normal and abnormal sensations and movements. Using a swab, an intraoral sensory examination can be performed to determine areas of hyposensitivity or hypersensitivity to tactile stimulation. The swab can be dipped in water of different temperatures or in flavorings and applied to various intraoral structures to map out the patient's responses. The information gained from this type of an examination can be useful in selecting food temperatures or flavors that promote preferred intraoral responses as well as in determining the most suitable locations for delivering these types of stimuli.

Frequently, a patient with a nasogastric tube demonstrates hyposensitivity to tactile stimulation in the oropharyngeal area surrounding the tube. Clinically, it appears that once this tube is removed, the patient is likely to regain sensory awareness in this immediate area. Decreased intraoral sensation is likely to contribute to a delayed swallow response, a problem commonly seen in patients who have sustained a brain injury.[2] It may be beneficial in certain cases to consider removing a nasogastric tube in the patient with profoundly decreased intraoral sensation and requesting that a more permanent surgical solution be used instead for supplemental nutrition. This may help to hasten the patient's return to safe oral intake.

Dentition

The therapist should check the overall condition of the teeth and determine whether any specific tactile or temperature sensitivities or problems exist. Facial injuries are quite common in this patient population and frequently involve some type of injury to the teeth. Problems with dentition may impede the patient's progression to more challenging food textures.

Tongue Control

In the normal swallowing processes, intraoral manipulation skills are essential for correct and timely positioning of the bolus into the posterior oral cavity. A great deal of strength and coordination are involved in these mechanics. Deficits in these areas will prolong the time required for the tongue to assist in shaping the bolus and positioning it so that it can trigger a swallow reflex.[12]

If capable of following commands, the patient can be asked to move the tongue laterally, protrude it forward, and elevate its posterior portion up toward the roof of the mouth. These motions can be assessed first without resistance, and then with resistance applied through a tongue blade. Tongue retraction can also be assessed, with resistance applied through the gloved hand of the examiner. The therapist should note the excursion of the patient's attempts, the presence of any asymmetries in movement, and the ability of the patient to rapidly change the direction of tongue motions. If capable of vocalizing, the patient may be asked to make sounds such as "la," "ta," "ka," or "ga," which encourage specific movements and coordination of the tongue. It may be necessary to simply assess passive mobility of the tongue in the low-level individual who cannot follow consistent commands for vocalization or movement. This is accomplished using a gloved hand or tongue blade to determine any resistance to passive movement.

Weaknesses in tongue control impair the formation and mobilization of the bolus in the intraoral cavity. The patient may tend to pocket food within the cheeks because of an inability of the tongue to reposition it back into the central bolus. Delayed intraoral transit time and poor bolus formation may cause some slippage of food into the pharynx before the triggering of a swallow reflex.

Progression of a feeding program to incorporate more challenging textures of food may be limited due to tongue weakness or endurance deficits.

Assessment of the Soft Palate and Posterior Pharyngeal Wall

Direct observation of the intraoral structures involved in the pharyngeal phase of swallowing can provide the therapist with important information regarding the efficiency of the patient's swallowing attempts. Pooling of secretions in the oropharynx may indicate problems with pharyngeal persistalsis and potential problems with aspiration. Food residue or secretions caked on any of the structures of the oropharynx may be indicative of decreased intraoral sensation.

The motion of both the soft palate and the posterior pharyngeal wall can be assessed reflexively or by asking for a volitional contraction of these structures. Assessment is best begun by observing the patient's own volitional efforts if possible. Active contraction of these structures can be seen if the patient is asked to forcefully vocalize an "ah" sound or to produce this sound using a high-pitched voice. Expected motion includes elevation and midline adduction of both the soft palate and posterior pharyngeal wall. Motion should be uniformly symmetrical. If the patient's effort produces a softly spoken sound, it will be difficult to appreciate much movement in these structures.

If volitional control of these structures cannot be assessed, a gag reflex can be elicited through tactile stimulation to the posterior third of the tongue, faucial arches, soft palate, or posterior pharyngeal wall. Some variability exists as to the optimal site for activation of this reflex, so it is important that the therapist try several areas within the oral cavity to promote the desired response. The gag response will produce elevation and adduction of the soft palate and posterior pharyngeal wall also. An assessment of these motions and the overall symmetry of the response should be made.

Decreased motion of the soft palate will prevent adequate closure of the nasopharynx during the pharyngeal swallow, thereby increasing the possibility of nasal reflux. The patient's speech may have a nasal quality to it as a result of the weakness seen here. Also, the therapist may notice that there is air leakage through the nose when the patient attempts to blow air out through the mouth. Decreased motion in the posterior pharyngeal wall may contribute to decreased pharyngeal peristalsis, with subsequent pooling of the bolus within the pharynx being likely. Markedly reduced sensation of these structures is likely to produce a delayed swallow reflex.

Laryngeal Control

Mobility and coordination are necessary for the larynx to meet the functional demands of swallowing. Approximately 1 inch of laryngeal elevation is required during a normal swallow to assure passage of the bolus through the pharynx and provide airway protection, thereby preventing aspiration.[9,10] A variety of assessments can be performed to determine this structure's capabilities. General passive mobility of the larynx can be assessed through gentle mobilization in the upward, downward, and lateral directions. Observation of the larynx during a spontaneous swallow is useful, with careful attention being paid to the amount of elevation that is noted. If vocalizations are possible, the patient can be instructed to perform a series of repetitive sounds such as "ah ah ah" spoken in a staccato manner. By assessing the crispness of these sounds, the therapist is able to determine whether laryngeal control is sufficiently functional to open and close the airway repetitively. Active movement and function of the larynx can also be assessed by asking the patient to change the pitch of his vocalizations from a low-sounding pitch to a high-sounding pitch. This exercise will promote elevation of the larynx if it is done properly. Difficulties in any of these areas may place the patient at risk for possible aspiration due to inefficient laryngeal mobility and coordination.

Assessment of a Patient's Cough

In a normal individual, a cough serves as a protective mechanism should aspiration occur. This mechanism is extremely important in a brain-injured patient, as cognitive and motor control deficits may make him a prime candidate for aspiration. Identifying the coughing capabilities of this patient population is critical in determining readiness for a feeding trial. Coughing attempts can be classified into three major categories.[13] A functional cough implies that the patient's coughing effort is capable of clearing the airway of any secretions. A weak functional cough implies that the attempt is effective for clearing the throat and for managing small amounts of secretions. A nonfunctional attempt implies that the patient is incapable of generating sufficient force to clear the airway of secretions. If a patient is capable of following commands, the therapist can ask the patient to cough volitionally. In listening to the coughing effort, the therapist must determine how effectively the patient is able to close off his glottis, as well as whether the effort was sufficiently forceful. Assessment of a reflexive cough is necessary in the patient who is unable to offer a volitional attempt. Observation of the patient by the therapist and other members of the rehabilitation team is necessary to develop a clinical impression of the adequacy of any reflexive coughing attempts. If frequent suctioning is required in a patient with a tracheostomy, the therapist is likely to be given ample opportunity to observe a reflexive cough.

To plan a treatment approach that will address coughing dysfunction effectively, the therapist should determine the factors that contribute to the etiology of this problem. If the patient has sufficient weakness affecting the muscles of inspiration, she may be incapable of taking in an adequate amount of air in the first part of the coughing attempt. The patient who has had sufficient respiratory problems since the onset of her brain injury is likely to display limitations in chest wall mobility that may further reduce her inspiratory efforts. The patient may also lack adequate abdominal muscle strength to generate a forceful expiration. It is common to find problems with adequate glottal closure in brain-injured patients; these may serve to further limit the force of their expiratory attempts.

SWALLOWING FLUOROSCOPY

A swallowing fluoroscopy is a useful examination for the brain-injured patient who presents with impaired intraoral, pharyngeal, or laryngeal control. This test is indicated especially when a tracheostomy tube is not present. Since many brain-injured patients may actually aspirate without reflexively coughing or clinically showing signs of distress, this test serves as an important adjunct to the physical examination of the patient.[2,14]

This test requires some active participation on the part of the patient and is therefore not indicated for the low-level individual. The patient should be positioned for the test just as he would be for a feeding trial. If the patient lacks adequate head and trunk control, he must be positioned on a table with a reclining back that can be adjusted to best suit his individual needs. The therapist determines the types of food consistencies to be tested and prepares the proper mixtures of barium paste or barium powder mixed with liquid. Thinner consistencies are aspirated more frequently, as they may move through the swallowing structures too quickly to stimulate a swallowing reflex.

During the actual fluoroscopy, the therapist introduces the barium and first evaluates the patient's swallowing response independent of any facilitative assistance. If needed, the therapist can then offer some facilitation of the swallowing attempt, either intraorally through some downward pressure on the tongue applied through a tongue blade or a quick stretch of the larynx to facilitate elevation. This will enable the therapist to see whether such facilitation is making a difference in the overall swallowing process. If the patient starts to aspirate and is capable of coughing volitionally, he should be encouraged to do so to see if in fact his efforts suffice to clear his airway. Similarly, any reflexive coughs that are performed can be evaluated for their efficacy in clearing the airway.

It must be remembered that the presence or absence of aspiration on a fluoroscopy trial may not necessarily be indicative of the patient's performance on all subsequent feeding trials. Should the therapist decide to initiate a feeding program based upon the patient's clinical assessment and fluoroscopy results, it is essential that the patient's clinical status continue to be monitored during and after each feeding trial to ensure the continued safety of these activities.

TREATMENT TECHNIQUES FOR MANAGING
SWALLOWING DYSFUNCTION

The techniques used in treating the swallowing deficits of the brain-injured patient are directed specifically at the problems identified through the therapist's evaluation. The overall success of any swallowing program is also dependent upon the therapist's ability to address the diversity of problems that influence the swallowing process, including pertinent physiologic, cognitive, and behavioral factors. Patient and family involvement and education are critical components of this endeavor, as is educating the entire rehabilitation team to the status and progress of the feeding program. The therapist must devise treatment plans that include a variety of techniques to prevent boredom on the part of the patient. Age-appropriate tasks must be chosen to improve patient acceptability and willingness to participate. The following section presents some ideas for managing those problems that were addressed in the previous section of this chapter.

Treating the Patient with Deficits in Head and Trunk Control

The physically involved patient with deficits in head and trunk control presents a significant challenge to the physical therapist. Clinically, postural control problems in these patients are generally related to difficulty in moving the pelvis into an anterior tilt position in sitting so as to create a stable base of support for the trunk and head.[15] The therapist addresses this issue by determining whether the etiology of this primary problem is related to limited range of lumbar extension or hip flexion, decreased motor control or awareness of the trunk, or abnormal trunk tone. If lumbar extension range is limited, the therapist can apply some mobilization techniques to improve mobility in sitting, followed by facilitation techniques to improve the patient's control within this new range of motion. A basic hip flexion stretch can be set up by positioning the patient on a tilt table and supporting one limb in a sling while the pelvis and contralateral limb are securely held against the table. Manual facilitation techniques can be used to promote an improved awareness of movement into an anterior tilt position with lumbar extension and to teach the patient how to deal with any possible abnormal trunk tone or motor control deficits. Once the therapist is better able to promote a stable base of support in sitting, it will be much easier to address the issues of inadequate thoracic and cervical extension using facilitative techniques.

Proper wheelchair positioning is crucial to promote ideal head and trunk postures, so that the structures involved in swallowing can be adequately treated. The addition of a solid seat and solid wheelchair back may be helpful in providing a firm support surface for the patient's pelvis and back. Lateral trunk supports may also be used to maintain trunk and head alignment over the base of support of the pelvis. A chest strap may be indicated for the patient who tends to fall forward or show a flexed trunk posture, something that is routinely seen if the patient has a tendency to cough frequently and forcefully due to possible aspiration or difficulty in clearing the airway. A recliner wheelchair reclined approximately 20 to 30° from upright may be used to position the head out of a forward flexed posture. The therapist may have to evaluate a variety of different commercially available head and neck supports if severe head control problems exist (see Ch. 6). All of these supports have their advantages and disadvantages, and must be evaluated carefully to best suit the patient's needs.

If the patient's head control deficits are too severe to allow for swallowing training to occur while the patient is upright in a wheelchair, then proper positioning in bed may be indicated. The head of the bed can be reclined slightly and neutral head and neck alignment attempted. It may be helpful to replace the patient's pillow with a folded towel so that the neck is not forced into excessive cervical flexion. Towel rolls may have to be placed along the sides of the patient's head to discourage excessive rotation. Education of other staff members, family, and visitors can be accomplished through the use of a clearly marked sign outlining the ideal bed positioning postures and procedures.

Dealing with Oral Defensiveness or Heightened Oral Reflexes

The goal of treatment of the orally defensive patient is to reduce his hypersensitivity to sensory stimuli through a gradual reintroduction of a variety of inputs. In using any desensitization techniques, the therapist must progress gradually to avoid overwhelming the patient with excessive amounts of stimulation delivered in too short a time. The patient is carefully observed to evaluate his response to each input. Abnormal facial posturing or movement away from the stimulus indicates that the patient perceives the stimulus as being too noxious. The patient's response to the stimulus may be delayed, so adequate time is needed to allow for this before the next stimulus is provided.

Gentle stroking of the perioral and surrounding facial areas with a soft cloth or applicator soaked in warm water is often a good starting activity for many patients with oral defensiveness or abnormal oral reflexes. As the patient begins to feel comfortable with this activity, the therapist can try using a different cloth with a rougher texture, like a washcloth. The temperature of the water can also be varied to provide an additional stimulus when the patient is ready to accept it.

Stroking the lips and the gums can also be accomplished with the use of an oral hygiene device such as a toothette. The soft, spongy tip of this device provides a good interface for beginning intraoral desensitization. Large swabs can be used to stroke over the gums and teeth in a slow and gentle manner. Some patients respond well to firm pressure applied to the lips through the application of the widest portion of a tongue blade held against them. Firm pressure applied over the masseter muscles may be useful in gaining relaxation in a patient who tends to demonstrate a bite reflex or grind his teeth excessively.

As the patient gradually responds to these desensitization techniques, the therapist will be able to enter the oral cavity with greater ease. This will allow further evaluation of the patient's intraoral function and the establishment of treatment goals directed at the entire swallowing process.

Promoting Improved Control of Oral-Phase Function

A great deal of creativity can be used in treating problems related to oral-phase control. Many of the treatment ideas can actually be used to manage more than one of the clinical deficits seen in this phase of the swallowing process. These techniques rely upon active participation on the part of the patient.

Problems with inadequate lip closure can be managed by applying either a quick ice or quick stretch technique to the perioral region, followed by a request for active movement to bring the lips together. A lighted candle or small, lightweight object can be the target of a blowing activity that will also facilitate lip closure. Blowing or sucking using a straw can also be used to address this problem.

Limitations in jaw opening frequently requires 15 to 20 minutes of static stretching using a number of stacked tongue blades placed between the upper and lower teeth.[11] This stretching exercise may have to be repeated several times a day, with the height of the pile of tongue blades being increased as tolerated. Inadequate jaw closure can be addressed by asking the patient to chew on a gauze-covered tongue blade or by applying manual resistance to a neck flexion effort.

Tongue mobility, strengthening, and coordination must be addressed in the patient experiencing lingual control deficits. If mobility is limited, the therapist can passively use a gloved hand to mobilize the tongue in a variety of directions to improve its range. This technique is also effective if an oral apraxia exists and the patient is unable to direct tongue movements on his own. The techniques of quick icing and quick stretching followed by active motion are effective in initiating movement. Resistance to active movement can be applied manually or through the use of a tongue blade as the patient is able to tolerate it. Active movement can be promoted through the same vocalization used in the initial patient assessment.

Dealing with Inadequate Function of the Soft Palate and Posterior Pharyngeal Wall

A variety of activities may be used to work on the problem of inadequate soft palate function. As indicated in the following text, many of these same activities can be used specifically to address decreased posterior pharyngeal wall control and intraoral sensory deficits.

Activities that involve blowing air through the mouth without allowing for nasal leakage will encourage soft palate control. Nasal leakage can be assessed by holding one finger under the patient's nose and feeling for air movement during the activity. The patient can be asked to blow on a feather, to blow a small lightweight ball across a table, or to blow on an object floating in water, such as a toy boat.

Blow bottles have been used quite successfully in the clinic to improve soft palate function. These are two bottles in a closed system that are interconnected, each with a separate blowing tube. Colored water is placed in one of the bottles, and the patient may either blow or suck this water into the adjoining bottle. Sucking the water from one bottle to the next presents a more challenging activity to the patient and can be incorporated progressively as the patient's soft palate function improves. Resisted sucking using this device is an excellent means of improving motor control deficits in the posterior pharyngeal wall also. This device works well with the brain-injured patient, as it entails an easily visible goal-directed task for the patient to complete.

Resisted neck flexion exercises tend to promote contraction of the soft palate and musculature of the posterior pharyngeal wall as well as the supra- and infrahyoid muscles. These exercises may serve several purposes in the patient's rehabilitation program in that they can be used to help promote functional skills such as learning to roll from supine to side lying and to promote head control in the physically involved patient.

Intraoral electrical stimulation is a technique that works well in the patient with markedly reduced sensation and motor control in the area of the soft palate and posterior pharyngeal wall. A standard portable stimulator that puts out a pulsatile current can be used for this purpose. The unit is set to deliver a current pulse that lasts approximately 4 seconds, followed by an off time of approximately 12 seconds. A long, slender adapter can be plugged into the stimulator's active lead hole. The adapter's tip acts as the active electrode and is initially placed on the patient's tongue while the amplitude of the stimulator is increased gradually until a contraction is elicited. The amplitude required to produce this contraction is usually a good starting amplitude for the soft palate and posterior pharyngeal wall musculature. The most effective motor points for the soft palate lie on either side of the uvula. The posterior pharyngeal wall presents with motor points on either side of the midline of this structure. The active electrode can be placed on one of these points, while the patient is asked to say "ah" as he feels the stimulation come on (Fig. 5-1). Many patients will be unable to comply with this request due to the overwhelming sensory deficits they are experiencing. This procedure is repeated approximately 10 times per treatment session, with rests given in between as needed. An electrical stimulation program may be used as a means of gauging the return of motor and sensory function within the mouth. Improved timing of the patient's own volitional response with the stimulated contraction may be gradually seen. As intraoral sensation improves, the patient may actually begin to perceive the electrical stimulation as a noxious stimulus. Increased sensitivity to a gag response may be another means of demonstrating patient progress intraorally and will also signal the therapist that the stimulation program is no longer an appropriate treatment option.

The heightened awareness of the soft palate or posterior pharyngeal wall gained through an intraoral electrical stimulation program can be followed up in the same treatment session with some other activities to further encourage active movement of these structures. For example, the therapist may use a

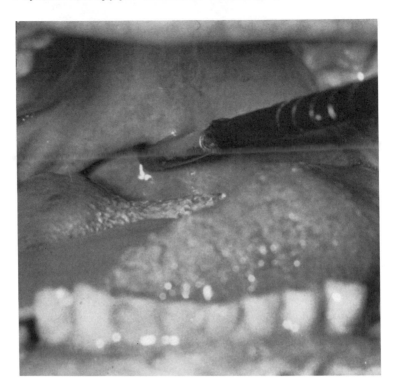

Fig. 5-1. A view inside of a patient's mouth illustrating the placement of the active electrode for electrical stimulation of the posterior pharyngeal wall. This picture was taken during the off cycle of the stimulation and shows the pharyngeal structures at rest. The patient's uvula is obscured by the position of the electrode.

swab dipped in cold water as a means of delivering a quick ice stimulus to the soft palate or posterior pharyngeal wall while asking for volitional movement through an "ah" vocalization.

Resisted tongue retraction using a gloved hand is another means of exercising the soft palate area and posterior pharyngeal wall musculature. Both of these structures are seen to contract in an effort to stabilize the posterior oral cavity as this activity is performed.

Treating Deficits in Laryngeal Control

The treatment of laryngeal deficits is generally directed at improving overall mobility of this structure or improving glottal closure capabilities. Many of the same techniques used in evaluating the function of the larynx can be incorporated in some way in the patient's treatment program.

Facilitation of laryngeal elevation can be accomplished by applying a quick stretch to the juxtalaryngeal area immediately before a swallow. As an alternative, quick ice can be delivered in this same area to heighten the patient's awareness of this structure and its intended movement. Gentle mobilization of the larynx may be helpful in some patients, especially if there appears to be some scarring at a closed tracheostomy site. Pitch change variations also tend to encourage laryngeal movement.

Vocalizations that incorporate a staccato sound are indicated for the patient with poor glottal closure. The patient should be instructed to make each sound as distinct as possible. Blowing activities that require controlled release of air are also useful in improving glottal closure skills. These can include blowing large bubbles in a controlled manner, slowly blowing out a candle, or blowing a light object slowly across a table. It may be helpful to have the patient practice his volitional cough skills if glottal closure problems limit expulsion pressures.

INITIATION AND PROGRESSION OF A FEEDING PROGRAM

The decision to initiate an oral feeding program in a brain-injured patient involves identifying whether some basic criteria have been met to ensure the patient's safety during swallowing.[9,10] A feeding trial is not initiated until the patient demonstrates at least weak intraoral manipulation skills. This ensures that the bolus can be properly positioned for its entry into the oropharynx. Weak functional control of the posterior pharyngeal wall is a prerequisite for movement of the bolus through the pharynx. A minimum of 1 inch of laryngeal elevation should be present to ensure adequate movement of this structure to prevent aspiration. The patient should also demonstrate at least weak functional cough abilities, either volitionally or reflexively, or should have a tracheostomy tube so that suctioning can be performed as needed. Medically, the patient must be clear of any active respiratory problems and should not be demonstrating evidence of aspiration. It is also important that the patient have adequate cognition to participate at least minimally in the feeding trial.

If a patient meets these basic criteria, the therapist may begin a feeding program. The consistency and amount of food that may be used in this program will vary depending on the patient's physical and cognitive deficits. Pureed consistencies of food are indicated for the patient who demonstrates intraoral manipulation problems, as these require the least muscular effort on the part of the tongue and intraoral musculature. This food consistency is also useful when dealing with the apraxic patient who lacks adequate coordination skills intraorally. If jarred baby foods are used, it may be helpful to add seasonings to them to improve their overall palatability. Information from the patient's family regarding his dietary likes and dislikes can be immensely helpful in ensuring success and interest at this stage of the feeding program. It may even be possible for the patient's family to bring in blenderized versions of some of his favorite foods. As the patient's chewing and manipulation skills improve, he may progress to a diet consisting of substances that are ground rather than pureed. Soft fruits and vegetables can also be included in this diet. The final goal of the swallowing program is to return the patient to regular foods whenever possible.

As the feeding program progresses, the therapist must make decisions related to the amount of oral intake the patient is capable of handling. Some factors that will influence the therapist's decision making include the amount of time the patient is able to attend to the task of eating, his muscular endurance for the process, and whether a significant amount of food can be handled within a reasonable time frame. The therapist should carefully monitor the exact amount of food the patient consumes in any one session. This information is essential for the dietitian as well as the nursing and medical staff following the patient's progress. If supplemental tube feeds are given, adjustments may have to be made so that adequate nutrition is provided to the patient at all stages of his swallowing program.

Liquids present a special challenge to the therapist involved in swallowing rehabilitation. Those untrained in swallowing dysfunction frequently feel a quick sip of water or other liquid could not possibly harm the patient and may comply with the patient's requests for a drink. Staff and family education is essential to ensure that problems will not arise as a result of others' good intentions. If the patient is experiencing difficulty handling liquids, a thickener can be added to the patient's favorite drink to make it easier for him to manage. The therapist must determine the best ratio of thickener to liquid to prevent possible aspiration.

It is frequently useful to apply a few drops of blue food coloring to the patient's food if he has a tracheostomy tube. If the patient should cough or need to be suctioned during or immediately after a feeding trial, it is very easy to detect if aspiration has occurred by looking for traces of the food coloring. This provides immediate feedback to the therapist as to the success or failure of that particular feeding trial.

If the patient is capable of self-feeding, the therapist must make sure that adequate supervision is provided at all times. Brain-injured patients frequently demonstrate poor self-monitoring of their oral intake; they are liable to place excessive amounts of food in their mouths or to rush through the swallowing process. The ideal setup involves the use of a quiet, distraction-free environment to maximize the patient's ability to attend to the task of eating. Poor judgment on the part of patients is likely to prevent them from recognizing any foods on their trays that are not of the prescribed consistency. It is therefore imperative that, in the inpatient setting, the patient's tray be carefully scrutinized as it arrives from the kitchen.

SUMMARY

Successful management of swallowing dysfunction in a brain-injured patient begins with a thorough evaluation of clinical deficits and the establishment of a treatment program that is directed at each of these problems. An interdisciplinary approach is required to promote carryover of specific positioning and feeding techniques and to ensure that the patient's dietary needs are met. Active involvement on the part of both patient and family is necessary for the safe progression of the feeding process.

REFERENCES

1. Winstein CJ: Neurogenic dysphagia: frequency, progression, and outcome in adults following head injury. Phys Ther 63:1992, 1983
2. Lazarus CL, Logemann JA: Swallowing disorders in closed head trauma patients. Arch Phys Med Rehabil 68:79, 1987
3. Cherney LR, Halper AS: Recovery of oral nutrition after head injury in adults. J Head Trauma Rehabil 4(4):42, 1989
4. Logemann JA: Evaluation and Treatment of Swallowing Disorders. College-Hill Press, San Diego, CA, 1983
5. Dobie RA: Rehabilitation of swallowing disorders. Am Fam Phys 17(5):84, 1978
6. Netter FH: Digestive System: Part I. Upper Digestive Tract. In The CIBA Collection of Medical Illustrations. Vol. 3. CIBA, New York, 1966
7. Heiden JS, Small R, Caton W, et al: Severe head injury: clinical assessment and outcome. Phys Ther 63:1946, 1983
8. Perry J, Nickel VL: Total cervical-spine fusion for neck paralysis. J Bone Joint Surg 41A(1):37, 1959
9. Winstein C: Evaluation and management of swallowing dysfunction. p. 39. In Professional Staff Association (eds): Rehabilitation of the Head Injured Adult: Comprehensive Physical Management. Rancho Los Amigos Hospital, Downey, CA, 1979
10. Stieger-Maguire C, Rushmore P: Dysphagia: evaluation and treatment. p. 32. In Professional Staff Association (eds): Stroke Rehabilitation: State of the Art 1984. Rancho Los Amigos Medical Center, Downey, CA, 1984
11. Hertling D, Kessler RM: Management of Common Musculoskeletal Disorders. 2nd Ed. J.B. Lippincott, Philadelphia, 1990
12. Lazarus CL: Swallowing disorders after traumatic brain injury. J Head Trauma Rehabil 4(4):34, 1989
13. Alvarez SE, Peterson M, Lunsford BR: Respiratory treatment of the adult patient with spinal cord injury. Phys Ther 61:1737, 1981
14. Logemann JA: Evaluation and treatment planning for the head-injured patient with oral intake disorders. J Head Trauma Rehabil 4(4):24, 1989
15. Fisher B: Effect of trunk control and alignment on limb function. J Head Trauma Rehabil 2(2):72, 1987

6 | Wheelchair Seating and Positioning

Mei Lee Chiu

A wheelchair seating "system" comprises an interrelated set of equipment components. When properly integrated, the individual components optimize the patients' quality of life by expanding opportunities for function in the home and community. This chapter provides a set of general guidelines used by physical therapists at Rancho Los Amigos Medical Center when prescribing wheelchairs and positioning systems for patients who have sustained a brain injury. This discussion is not a clinical protocol. The most reliable means of providing safe and functional seating systems is not derived from protocols but, rather, from problem-based solutions, experimentation, and sound clinical judgment.

This chapter presents an overview of benefits for seating and considerations for evaluation and wheelchair selection. A discussion of positioning principles includes suggestions for equipment components that address specific positioning problems. The significance of the trunk posture and alignment is prominent in much of the discussion about positioning principles. The positional and functional relationships that exist between the trunk, head, and extremities are used to guide clinical decisions that extend beyond the impact of hands-on therapy. The seating system described here is just one aspect of the therapeutic continuum. Therapy does not end when the therapist's hands are removed and the client is returned to the wheelchair. The wheelchair is considered an extension of therapy as it preserves functional goals achieved by the patient under the therapist's guidance.

BENEFITS OF OPTIMIZING SEATING INTERVENTION

Meeting the seating needs of brain-injured patients and their caregivers involves a comprehensive management approach. There is wide diversity within the patient population. At one end of the spectrum are patients with cognitive

117

impairment and few physical limitations. These patients may require constant supervision for safety and little if any physical assistance. A wheelchair may be used in the community as a constraint, if not restraint, by the caregiver. At the other end of the spectrum are patients with significant physical restrictions whose primary lifestyle is focused upon the wheelchair. These patients require an extensive system of equipment components to optimize wheelchair tolerance. Between the two extremes are various types of patients, each with an array of unique cognitive and physical considerations.

Properly positioning patients who have sustained brain injury in appropriate wheelchairs offers several important benefits. Three of the most important advantages are optimizing level of alertness, providing pressure relief, and facilitating trunk stability and functional mobility. In addition to its contribution to cognitive and physical function, the wheelchair plays an important role in offering opportunities to interact with the environment, thereby fulfilling important social and psychological needs of the client and the caregivers.

Prolonged periods of time in bed alter the level of alertness in patients with low cognitive function. A patient functioning at LOC III (Rancho Los Amigos Levels of Cognitive Functioning Scale) may be somewhat confused by the images he or she perceives by viewing the world from a horizontal position in bed. This alteration in space orientation may contribute to periods of impaired attention and interaction with the environment. At this stage of recovery, a patient functioning at LOC III reacts slowly and inconsistently; therefore, he or she should be placed in an environment that is free from distractions and facilitates optimal cognitive improvement. Positioning this patient in a wheelchair reduces time spent in bed and encourages vertical orientation. The upright position stimulates a number of sensory systems, including the visual, proprioceptive, and vestibular systems.

Another benefit of seating intervention is ensuring comfort and alleviating excessive pressures. Persistent decubitus ulcers limit wheelchair sitting tolerance and significantly increase overall medical costs. Risk factors for skin breakdown include the amount of soft tissue present, sensory status, ability to perform pressure relief in the chair, etc. While no one wheelchair or seat cushion guarantees against the detrimental effects of excessive sitting pressures, patients and caregivers must be educated in preventive measures and the consequences of inconsistent follow-through with pressure-relieving techniques. To maintain adequate distribution of seating pressures, clinicians and caregivers must learn to assess continuously the appropriateness of the placement and function of all positioning devices. As time passes, seating components must be changed and modified as warranted by variations in the patient's weight or sitting tolerance.

Finally, proper wheelchair positioning is a critical factor in achieving a balance between (1) positioning for stability and (2) optimizing functional mobility. The wheelchair and seating components are used to position the patient in the midline and to form a stable base of support for the rest of the body. A stable trunk and pelvis complex is the foundation by which an individual accesses the extremities for functional activities and interacts with the environment.

Stabilization of the proximal body segments (i.e., the trunk and pelvis) is a key principle in seating the client who has sustained brain injury. This principle is discussed in greater detail below.

THE COMPREHENSIVE ASSESSMENT

Seating and positioning are influenced by several aspects of the evaluation. A thorough assessment includes these five areas: the client's medical status, functional range of motion, cognitive status, visual and perceptual deficits, and movement dysfunction. The integration of these five aspects into the problem solving schema guides the selection of positioning equipment.

Specific seating solutions may be dictated by the patient's medical status. For example, a reclining or tilt feature may be prescribed for patients exhibiting poor endurance, compromised respiratory function, high risk for skin breakdown, or orthostatic hypotension. These patients require frequent changes in position to maximize sitting tolerance. While optional positioning may be beneficial to some individuals, it may not be helpful to other patients. Reclining or tilting the patient's back alters orientation in space and visual perception; it may also position the patient negatively for speech or swallowing.

Functional range of motion (ROM) is the range required at various joints to allow performance of specific activities with ease and efficiency. Determining the nature of the deformity and its temporary or permanent influence on the body is crucial in addressing this problem. A ''flexible'' deformity is one that is correctable, while a ''fixed'' deformity does not respond to manual positioning techniques. The seating system should (1) correct and stabilize a flexible deformity and (2) accommodate and stabilize a fixed deformity.

A flexible deformity can be corrected with positioning equipment, manual adjustment, or a short-term serial casting program. For example, a client with muscular imbalance in the trunk develops a flexible scoliosis (Fig. 6-1). By gently realigning the curvatures, the clinician is able to correct the deformity manually. With the help of several positioning components, the trunk is aligned in the wheelchair and the flexible scoliosis is thus corrected (Fig. 6-2).

By contrast, a ''fixed'' deformity is not correctable with these treatment techniques. If surgery is not indicated for such a chronic orthopedic problem, the seating system must accommodate the fixed deformity. In the case of a fixed scoliosis, seating components are used to accommodate the trunk position, prevent further deterioration, and maximize comfort and function (Fig. 6-3).

Selection of equipment is also influenced by the patient's cognitive status, including attention span, behavior, and memory. For example, a patient functioning at LOC IV may demonstrate confusion and poor frustration tolerance, requiring removal of the armrests in favor of supporting the arms only with pillows. While specific arm supports may be warranted at that point in time, clinical judgment indicates that it is not in the best interest of the patient to use extraneous positioning tools with straps and buckles because of their role

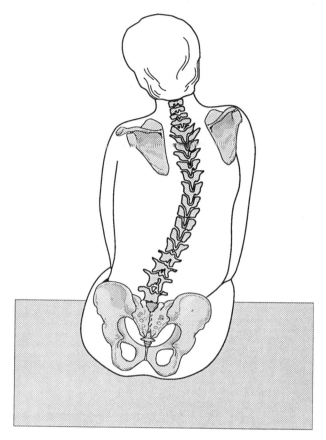

Fig. 6-1. Flexible scoliosis.

in distracting the patient and contributing to his or her frustration. Pillows are not ideal support devices, but they may be beneficial during this state of heightened confusion and frustration.

The presence of visual and perceptual problems may guide selection of specific positioning tools. For example, a patient demonstrating hemianopia or visual neglect of one side of the body and environment requires specific consideration to optimize safety in the chair. If the patient's orientation in space is altered, sturdy positioning aids and belts may be required to ensure safety during wheelchair mobility and discourage the client from transferring from the chair unnecessarily. The paretic arm may be secured to the armrest to prevent slipping, and bright colors may be applied to help the patient identify wheel locks and brakes. A patient demonstrating problems with depth perception may have difficulty with transfers if he or she has trouble distinguishing between objects in the visual field.

Assessment of movement dysfunction integrates all four of the aforemen-

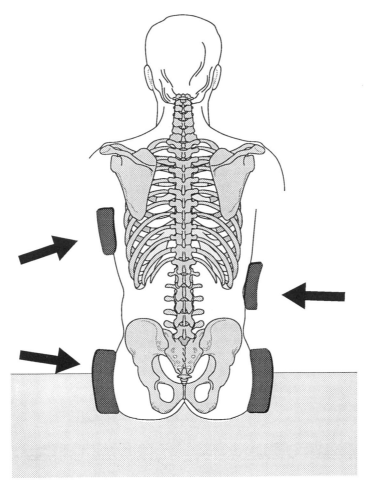

Fig. 6-2. Positioning equipment (with three points of support) corrects a flexible scoliosis.

tioned aspects of the evaluation and draws upon other neurologic influences to render a dynamic and functional picture of the client. Movement is produced by an interaction of several systems inherent in the body, including the motor, sensory, perceptual, and balance systems. While the specific contribution of each system to the production of movement is not known, these systems collaborate to produce the desired end product: effective and efficient movement to accomplish a particular functional task.

Movement dysfunction is defined as impairment of one's ability to carry out the desired movement pattern proficiently. A patient with neurologic deficits from a brain injury often demonstrates deficiencies in his or her ability to move specific body segments or the entire body. Movement is produced from a coordinated interplay of factors within a multidimensional system rather than

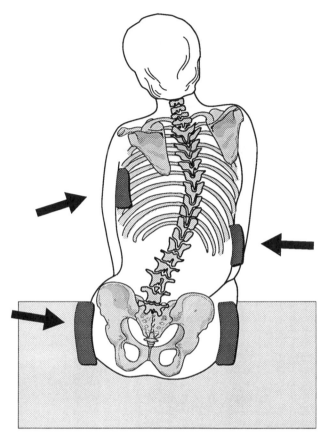

Fig. 6-3. Positioning equipment prevents further progression of a fixed scoliosis.

merely as motions at isolated joints. Movement dysfunction must then be observed as it relates to functional tasks rather than as isolated joint activity. For example, asking a patient with neurologic impairment to bring the paretic hand up to the head provides some information about upper extremity movement through space. However, this task would have more functional significance if the patient were asked to use a hairbrush. An analysis of this second task yields more substantive information about movement that incorporates the influences of static and sustained muscle activity (holding the hairbrush) and dynamic and sustained muscle activity (moving the arm against gravity, upper extremity sensory/proprioceptive feedback, etc.)

Movement dysfunction may be influenced by the presence of spasticity, dynamic muscle spasms, associated reactions, and abnormal movement patterns. The relationship of these factors to each other and their role in movement and alignment are the basis of much clinical discussion. Trunk alignment and the positional relationship of body segments to each other play a major role in influencing motor control and abnormal posturing. Understanding the factors that contribute to movement dysfunction helps to guide the selection of seating equipment to optimize alignment of all body segments, reduce abnormal movement patterns and provide a stable base of support for functional activities.

SELECTION OF THE WHEELCHAIR AND SEATING SYSTEM

Selecting the wheelchair and seating components requires creative integration and application of several factors. During the selection process, clinicians are challenged to thoughtfully consider the restrictions imposed by the funding source or third-party payer, social factors and individual preference, and the clinical findings described above. Clear-cut solutions for all seating problems may not be easily available. Every positioning system offers different benefits and disadvantages. The "best" systems are derived from a series of clinical trials with various components. The end product may consist of a series of compromises, integrating function with cost, convenience, practicality, and individual preference.

Key to the prescription of many seating systems is the funding source. In today's health care environment, third-party payers responsible for authorizing funds for patient equipment are scrutinizing prescriptions and limiting funds for medical equipment. Therefore clinicians are held accountable for articulating the patient's needs skillfully and educating the third-party payers on the principles and rationale upon which sound clinical decisions are based. Clinicians must be proficient in their documentation and employ such strategies as including photographs with their equipment prescriptions to adequately support the medical justification. As the health care delivery system changes and evolves, the status of funds for medical equipment will continue to be an issue of concern for health care providers. The scope of seating system options may be increasingly restricted, as reducing expenditure continues to be the prevailing theme. If funding from third-party payers is not available, it may be necessary to investigate nontraditional means of funding (such as charitable donations) or to develop creative low-cost seating systems in the clinic.

Several aspects—including the home and social environment, support network, cultural factors, and individual preference—contribute to the patient/caregivers' acceptance of the wheelchair and the seating system. Awareness and integration of these issues guide the clinician in thoughtfully educating the patient and caregivers and in soliciting support for clinical decisions regarding equipment selection. For example, social acceptance by the peer group may influence a young patient's decision to accept or reject a particular wheelchair system. This issue and others may restrict a clinician's equipment selection options. Clinicians must also consider that equipment issued with the best intentions is frequently rejected if it is not practical or simple to use, easily accepted and assimilated by the social support system, and readily maintained and assembled for routine use.

Finally, the clinician must integrate the benefits of seating intervention and the evaluation findings into the concept that the wheelchair is an adjunct to the therapeutic program. The clinician spends much effort in therapy trying to facilitate motor control, enhance trunk alignment, optimize mobility, and maximize function. This hands-on treatment time is merely a fraction of the total time that the patient spends in the wheelchair. If the wheelchair is seen as an extension of the therapy program, the efforts spent on hands-on treatment would be more effectively utilized. The chair should be used to maintain the gains achieved with hands-on therapy: preserve ROM, utilize motor control, and enhance functional tasks such as eating at the table and crossing the legs when tying shoelaces.

Cognitive and physical deficits may also guide the clinical decision toward or away from power wheelchairs. Powered wheelchair mobility is reserved for a select population of patients for whom manual wheelchair mobility is not a feasible option because of significant endurance problems, cardiac/respiratory complications, or impaired motor control. Clinicians must be strict with the following selection criteria to ensure safe mobility in the community: Power wheelchair users must be free of significant visual and perceptual deficits and must demonstrate adequate motor function, sitting tolerance, and control of dynamic spasms (e.g., myoclonus). These patients should function consistently at or above LOC VI.

There are numerous and continuous technological advances in the field of seating and rehabilitation equipment. A valuable group of consultants includes medical equipment vendors, equipment manufacturers, and seating specialists at large rehabilitation centers. These consultants can offer comparative information regarding cost, durability, and patient/clinician preference. Seating specialists are often therapists or other health care providers who can offer a clinical perspective on the seating system's influence on overall functional ability.

THE SIGNIFICANCE OF TRUNK ALIGNMENT

It is necessary to discuss anatomic relationships and address the contribution of the trunk to optimal wheelchair positioning. References to the trunk in this discussion include both the upper trunk (scapulae, cervical and thoracic spine) and the lower trunk (lumbar spine and pelvis). The trunk plays such a significant role because it is the body's primary point of stability. A stable trunk complex acts as the foundation for a well-balanced base of support and is the basis of functional mobility of the head and extremities.

A review of anatomy reveals that the posture of the spine consists of three balanced curves: cervical lordosis, thoracic kyphosis, and lumbar lordosis (Fig. 6-4). The spine is an unbroken chain. Any changes in one segment of that chain leads to compensatory changes in all the spinal curves. Figure 6-5 shows that posterior tilt of the pelvis on the sitting surface leads to flexion of the entire spine and a forward head position. This relationship points to an important functional implication for wheelchair patients. Specifically, malalignment or restricted mobility in one area of the trunk affects the entire trunk. Likewise,

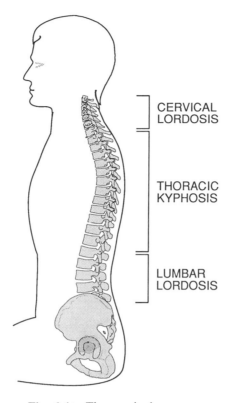

Fig. 6-4.   Three spinal curves.

CERVICAL
LORDOSIS

THORACIC
KYPHOSIS

LUMBAR
LORDOSIS

correcting one postural deviation may affect more than one area of the trunk. For example, when the patient with impaired motor control in Figure 6-5 is placed in an appropriate wheelchair seat with a positioning belt and lumbar pad, the position of the head also changes as the seating components realign the trunk over the pelvis (Fig. 6-6). One of the first goals that a clinician must achieve with a wheelchair and seating system is correction of postural deviations of the trunk and alignment of the spinal curves.

The significance of a stable base of support has functional implications for all individuals who must function from a chair, whether it is a desk chair or a wheelchair. A proper support base in the chair allows other body structures to be used effectively in carrying out activities efficiently within the base of support (e.g., eating at the table), outside the base (reaching forward for an object on the ground), and around the base and across midline (reaching around to pull a shirt across the opposite shoulder). An individual is able to perform these and other more complicated tasks most effectively when the support base is stable and steady.

Generally, a broader base of support offers several advantages over a narrower one. Normally in the wheelchair, the weight-bearing surfaces include the buttocks, thighs, feet, and sometimes the hands and forearms. When the sup-

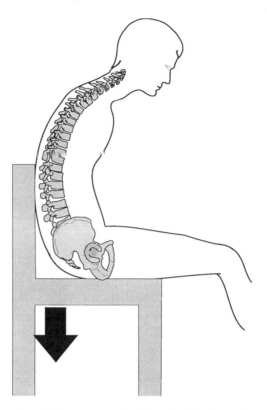

Fig. 6-5. Posterior pelvic tilt is associated with spinal flexion. Body weight falls behind the ischial tuberosities.

port base encompasses a larger area, body weight can be distributed proportionately to all these surfaces. This weight distribution also transfers sitting pressures and minimizes excessive pressure under the ischial tuberosities and the sacrum. In addition, a broader support base is generally more stable than a narrow base (e.g., standing with a wider stance is more stable than standing with the feet close together).

Figure 6-5 illustrates that a significant amount of weight falls behind the ischial tuberosities when an individual sits in a position of extreme trunk flexion. The support base is limited to the buttocks region, while the upper and lower extremities are not actively functioning as part of the base of support. Since the support base is narrow, the individual is less stable in this position. A functional activity such as prolonged wheelchair propulsion would be difficult. The upper extremities must work harder to propel the chair forward because (1) so much of the body weight falls behind the pelvis, (2) this position of excessive upper trunk flexion limits functional upper extremity mobility, and (3) the forward head position limits visual range. Figure 6-7 indicates that once the trunk is realigned properly over the pelvis, the entire base of support

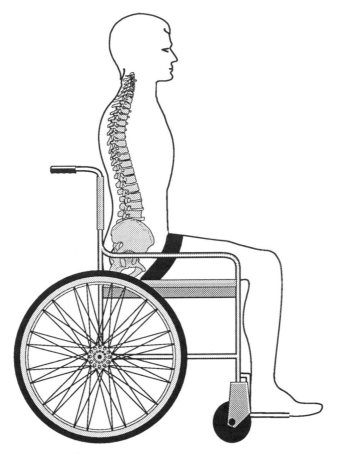

Fig. 6-6. An appropriate wheelchair and seating system aligns the trunk over the pelvis and the base of support.

changes; weight is borne more directly by the ischial tuberosities, thighs, and feet. Wheelchair propulsion is performed with less difficulty than before because extension of the upper trunk increases upper extremity mobility and the position of the head increases visual perception.

SETTING UP THE SYSTEM

Setting up a wheelchair system requires thoughtful incorporation of all the principles and considerations mentioned in the foregoing discussions. A prevailing theme in this section relates back to the previous references to the postural relationship between the trunk and the head/extremities. Deviations in alignment and movement dysfunction may be closely related; therefore a solution for one component may positively affect the other component. While

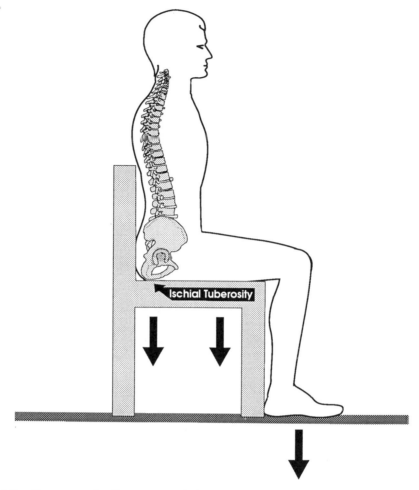

Fig. 6-7. Proper trunk alignment optimizes weight distribution, as indicated by the arrows pointing downward.

the wheelchair seating system is just one aspect of the entire therapeutic program, it has far-reaching implications.

Finding the "best" seating system to meet the unique needs of each patient requires creative problem-solving skills and the freedom to mix and match components. Assessment and management are interdependent. When the clinician evaluates and observes the patient under different conditions, he or she generates assumptions about the possible causes and effects of various postural deviations. As the clinician tries different components to correct the deformities, these evaluation assumptions and management solutions are either validated or refuted. By maintaining the problem-solving frame of reference, the clinician learns from each assessment/management trial and makes appropriate modifications to the seating system as new knowledge is gained.

Most home and office chairs are padded and constructed of solid foundations. Manufacturers meticulously design home and office furniture to maximize comfort and endurance for long periods of sitting. A chair that is "too comfortable" (e.g., a director's folding canvas chair) does not promote optimal sitting tolerance. Wheelchair patients must be given this same consideration because of the functional expectations placed upon them. Comfort and endurance in the chair become basic issues of survival for these patients. The first step in setting up the system is replacement of the sling seat and back in the existing wheelchair. Sling upholstery stretches over time, encouraging poor trunk alignment and contributing to excessive trunk flexion. By replacing the sling upholstery with a solid seat and back, a firm base is provided for the patient. An appropriate cushion is then placed on top of the sturdy plastic or wooden base. The discussion that follows assumes that a solid seat and back are placed in each wheelchair.

The Trunk

The torso is divided into the upper trunk (scapulae, cervical spine, thoracic spine, and all the muscular attachments) and the lower trunk (lumbar spine, pelvis, and the attached muscles). The trunk is optimally situated at a "neutral" position. Figure 6-7 illustrates that neutral trunk posture is an erect balanced position with slight anterior pelvic tilt and equal weight bearing on both ischial tuberosities. This discussion will focus on the following trunk and pelvic deviations: (1) trunk flexion and posterior pelvic tilt and (2) lateral lean/scoliosis and pelvic obliquity. Chronic positioning in these positions may result in disproportionate weight distribution and decubitus ulcers, compromised respiratory function with restriction of the thoracic cavity, and impaired visual perception as the head follows the curve of the upper trunk.

Trunk flexion and posterior pelvic tilt are common positioning problems among patients who have sustained a brain injury. This results from weakness, prolonged bed rest, and habitual premorbid positioning. These patients are often observed sliding forward and out of the wheelchair seat. To keep the trunk erect against the solid back, the pelvis must be stabilized against the back by placing a positioning belt low on the pelvis or across the upper aspect of the thighs (Fig. 6-6). Placing the belt too high across the pelvis offers inadequate support by facilitating hip extension and encouraging the patient to slide farther forward (Fig. 6-8).

Lateral trunk lean and scoliosis are discussed together because their clinical manifestations are similar. Pelvic obliquity is asymmetrical elevation of one side of the pelvis in relation to the opposite side and may be associated with either of these trunk postures. The difference between a fixed and a flexible scoliosis is discussed above under the "A Comprehensive Assessment." A three-point control system (as depicted in Figs. 6-2 and 6-3) is most effective in maintaining the desired trunk position. Supports placed on either side of the trunk are used to counterbalance lateral deviation. Since the hips and pelvis

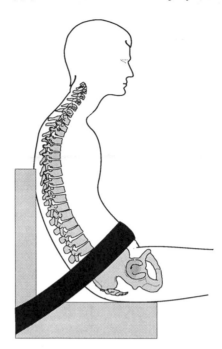

Fig. 6-8. Incorrect placement of positioning belt for patient with tendency to slide forward.

often shift laterally when the trunk is flexed, placing thigh supports on either side of the pelvis helps to alleviate this problem and maintain midline orientation of the pelvis. A flexible pelvic obliquity may be eliminated as the trunk is realigned with seating equipment. If a pelvic obliquity is still present, it may be necessary to use a foam seat cushion to balance the pelvic asymmetry. This is accomplished using a 3- to 4-inch firm cushion with the section directly under the elevated side cut out to a depth of 1 to 2 inches and replaced with softer foam. This technique allows the elevated side to sink down into the foam cushion and balances the deviation (Fig. 6-9).

The Head and Neck

Correct positioning of the head and neck is fundamental to human interaction. Swallowing, eye contact, and speech production are enhanced when the head is aligned properly over the trunk. Finding the most appropriate support may require several trial sessions. The following are guidelines to consider when evaluating various commercially available head supports.

The purpose of the head support is to place the head and neck in a position of comfort, functional mobility, and adequate stability.

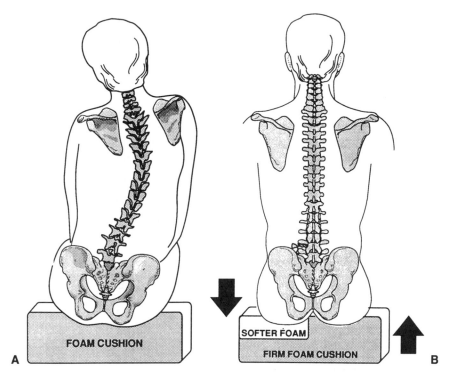

Fig. 6-9. (**A**) A spinal curve with pelvic obliquity unaccommodated on a standard foam cushion. (**B**) A custom foam cushion re-aligns a flexible spine and pelvis over the base of support.

Supporting the occiput provides stability and minimizes fatigue of the neck muscles.

Head supports with lateral projections may cause discomfort against the temples and pinch the ears.

Rubbing against the padded surfaces may cause shearing and excessive pressure on the scalp. Covering the head support with a "sheepskin" or satin material diminishes the risk of skin breakdown.

The head support should not obstruct vision.

There may be a number of patients for whom a standard support device does not adequately position the head. Such patients may include those with very poor endurance, spasticity of the neck flexors, skin breakdown due to excessive rubbing against the head support, or those with severe cognitive impairment. In this case, the standard head support may be replaced or augmented by a soft cervical collar. This device is made for minor neck injuries and not for the purpose of positioning the head. It should not be considered a positioning tool of choice but may be used temporarily while other options are being considered. Since the mandible is not a weight-bearing surface, prolonged use of a chin support may cause orthodontic complications, such as symptoms associated with temporomandibular joint dysfunction.

Finally, a strap (sometimes called a "halo" strap) may be used to provide anterior support for a patient with a chronic forward head position. Attached to the head support, this strap is placed at the level of the forehead to maintain proper head position against the head support device. The strap is not consistently effective with all patients as it has a tendency to slip, sometimes covering the patient's eyes. If long-term positioning of the forward head with a support device is unsuccessful, it may be necessary to place the patient in a slightly reclined wheelchair.

The Hip Joint

The ideal sitting position for most activities of daily living is an upright trunk with approximately 80 to 90° of hip flexion. This position maximizes weight bearing through the buttocks, thighs, and feet. Ideal hip position also includes neutral rotation and abduction/adduction of the femurs. Because of their attachment to the lower trunk, the position of the femurs directly affects trunk alignment. For example, excessive hip abduction in a patient with an unsupported trunk facilitates trunk flexion/posterior pelvic tilt and results in a tendency to slide forward in the seat. This discussion will focus on the following deviations: hip joint angle greater than or less than 90°, abducted and externally rotated femurs, adducted and internally rotated femurs, and "windswept" deformity.

A hip joint angle above 90° of flexion may be considered as excessive hip flexion. This position may be caused by contractures or spasticity of the hip or trunk flexors. The seat may be angled into flexion with a "wedge" seat. The purpose of the seat is to position the knees higher than the level of the hips; this is accomplished by angling the solid seat or cutting out a foam cushion at the desired angle. A positioning belt is used to secure the pelvis to the back of the seat. It may be more difficult to transfer the patient from the seat because the pelvis is so securely stabilized in it. In addition, a patient exhibiting severe extensor spasticity or myoclonus may be placed in a wedge to inhibit these abnormal movements. The degree of appropriate seat angulation must be determined by clinical trial. The clinician must balance between (1) excessive hip flexion, which may cause excessive trunk and head/neck flexion, and (2) inadequate hip flexion, which will not sufficiently inhibit spasticity.

A hip joint angle below 90° may be present as a result of contractures or spasticity of the hip or trunk extensors. The most feasible means of positioning such a patient is reclining the back of the wheelchair to the angle of the hip joint restriction and securing the pelvis with a positioning belt.

Femurs positioned in excessive adduction and internal rotation may occur when the footrests are placed too low for adequate limb support or as a result of spasticity of the associated muscles. Positioning solutions include a sturdy seat cushion to support the weight-bearing surfaces and proper adjustment of the footrests. Utilizing medial thigh supports or straps to prevent further adduction requires extreme caution because of the potential for skin breakdown.

Another common problem is femurs positioned in excessive abduction and external rotation. The lateral aspect of the thighs may rub against the metal wheelchair frame, causing discomfort and skin breakdown. The posture may be attributed to a wheelchair that is too wide for the patient, footrests placed too high for adequate limb support, or imbalance of the hip musculature. Seating solutions include fitting the patient with an appropriate wheelchair, proper adjustment of the footrest height, and placing support pads along the lateral aspects of the thighs to ensure neutral alignment of each femur.

An asymmetrical deviation called the "windswept" deformity occurs when one thigh is abducted/externally rotated and the other is adducted/internally rotated. Both knees are essentially pointing in the same direction. The trunk may present with a compensatory postural deformity. There may also be a compensatory component of trunk asymmetry. Positioning solutions for this complicated set of postural deviations include a combination of the options mentioned above. As each femur is aligned and secured properly, the feet should also be secured to the footrests to ensure that they remain in a weight-bearing position and help to guide the direction of the femurs.

The Lower Extremities

The lower extremities are significant to the overall seating scheme because of their role in contributing to the stable base of support. The optimal lower extremity weight-bearing position includes plantigrade placement of the feet on the footrests, neutral ankle and subtalar joint positions, and the knees positioned at or slightly below the level of the hips.

Knee positioning problems include difficulty achieving adequate knee flexion or extension range because of spasticity or contractures. In some cases, lower extremity positioning splints may be used to maintain the desired knee and ankle position while the patient is in the wheelchair. When the standard footrests and elevating leg rests do not provide adequate support to the legs, it may be necessary to custom-fabricate leg supports in the clinic. Custom fabrication may involve using a combination of materials including foam, straps, wood, hard plastic, and so on. The overall goals for positioning the lower legs should complement the goals for aligning the femurs and feet.

The ankle joint position is significant in its relationship to the weight-bearing surfaces of the feet. Optimal weight bearing through the soles of the feet can best be accomplished when the feet are plantigrade against a flat surface. When the upper body moves on the seat surface, as when the patient reaches forward for an object, weight is shifted from the ischial tuberosities forward to the feet while the patient's trunk moves forward. When the feet are not properly placed on the floor or the footrests, upper extremity functional activity and trunk stability are significantly compromised.

Equinus or equinovarus are common ankle problems that interfere with positioning the feet on the footrests. Assessment of the patient's movement and movement dysfunction helps to determine whether the deformity occurs in isolation or as part of a lower extremity abnormal movement pattern. The ankle/foot orthosis and shoe holder are two devices that may be used to position a mild ankle deformity. The ankle/foot orthosis is used to position the distal lower extremity for several activities, including wheelchair sitting and ambulation. The orthosis corrects the equinus or equinovarus position and places the ankle joint in the desired position on the footrest. A shoe holder is a hard plastic plate that is fastened to the footrest. The foot is then held in place on the shoe holder with a series of straps. If the deviation is relatively mild and the deformity is flexible, the patient may respond well to an orthotic device, the shoe holder, or a combination of both.

A severe abnormal movement pattern of the lower extremity or a fixed ankle deformity significantly limits the weight-bearing capabilities of the lower extremities. The movement pattern of these extremities must be addressed as a whole; successful positioning of such an extremity requires the application of stabilizing forces from both the proximal and distal ends of the extremity. Once the proximal lower extremity is stabilized, the distal portion may respond well to the ankle/foot orthosis and shoe holder. If the ankle deformity is fixed and cannot be positioned in these devices, a custom leg splint may be used to accommodate the deviation by protecting against skin breakdown and preventing further loss of range.

The Upper Extremities

Prescribing upper extremity positioning equipment for patients who have sustained brain injury offers a unique learning experience. Each patient's neurologic sequelae presents unique features that occur in isolation or as a pattern of events. Management of a flaccid arm with no ROM limitations varies significantly from management of an upper extremity with severe spasticity, muscle imbalance, and ROM limitations. Positioning components must address the stability and mobility needs required for optimal upper extremity function.

A comprehensive management approach considers the relationship between the trunk and the upper extremities. A review of biomechanical principles reveals that normal upper extremity activity derives in part from proper alignment and stability of the trunk. A stable trunk forms the foundation for functional mobility of the scapulae on the thorax. Moreover, stability of these proximal body structures sets up a mechanical advantage for the humerus to move through space functionally and effectively. Deficiencies in these key components further compromises the patient who already exhibits impaired motor control.

A flaccid upper extremity requires adequate support at all times to minimize edema and to decrease its potential for injury. A problem commonly associated with a flaccid upper extremity is shoulder subluxation. This is an alteration in the suprahumeral space. The suprahumeral space is formed by the articular space between the head of the humerus, the coracoid process, and the overhanging acromion. Subluxation is attributed to several factors including (1) lack of motor control about the shoulder girdle, disrupting the positional relationship of the structures in the suprahumeral space, (2) lack of mobility between the humerus and the structures of the trunk, and (3) impaired mobility between the scapula and the thorax.

A comprehensive management program to reduce the subluxation begins with constant support of the shoulder in the wheelchair to reduce pain and prevent further stretching of the joint capsule and all the muscular attachments. There are many commercially available support devices to support the flaccid upper extremity. The height adjustment of these arm supports must be considered, because incorrect height adjustment further aggravates the symptoms. An arm support that is too low may provide insufficient support for the shoulder and further stretch the soft tissues, while a support that is placed too high for the patient forces the humeral head into the glenoid fossa at an undesirable angle. Finally, a flexible strap may be used to secure the upper extremity in the desired position on the arm support. Placing a strap across the dorsal aspect of the hand, rather than across the forearm or elbow, secures the upper extremity while the forearm is unrestrained and the elbow is free to flex and extend as the patient leans forward and laterally during functional activities in the wheelchair.

The influence of spasticity, dynamic spasms, or abnormal movement patterns often presents a complicated positioning dilemma. Key to the prescription of equipment solutions for this group of clients is familiarity with the neurologic sequelae and an ongoing assessment/management process. Patients with severe abnormal movement patterns may have limited success with restrictive positioning components. These patients present with such limited range, severe dynamic spasms, or limited tolerance to positioning devices that forcing the upper extremity into arm supports is counterproductive. Some of these individuals may be well positioned at rest but exhibit such strong associated reactions during a cough or yawn that the upper extremities pull away from the arm supports. When standard arm supports are not effective, it may be necessary to use custom splints for hand positioning and support the forearms on a padded lapboard. Placing the arms on a lapboard decreases the potential for skin breakdown but does not hold the upper extremities in place during an associated reaction or abnormal movement pattern. When the abnormal movements occur, the arms may require repositioning on the lapboard.

Patients with mild/moderate spasticity or abnormal movement patterns may be functional with commercially available support devices. Some arm supports offer a positioning strap or a hand piece fashioned in the shape of a "dome" or "cone." These positioning features should be carefully assessed over a period of time. In some cases, these accessories are beneficial. In other situations, these arm support features may increase the abnormal movement pattern because the shape or placement of the arm support imposes a stretch on the spastic muscles. Selection of the arm support begins with an assessment of the dynamic range available in the upper extremity. As the patient and clinician move the arm through space, the clinician observes the range limitations at all the joints in the upper extremity, and notes the influence of the upper trunk alignment. Variations in trunk alignment and upper extremity positioning as the arm and hand are placed on the lap, on various arm supports, and so on are also noted. This guides the selection of support devices because the clinician must choose optimum placement of the arm support at a location that minimizes spasticity/abnormal movement patterns, enhances proper trunk alignment, and maximizes functional mobility of the other body structures.

SUMMARY

Setting up a wheelchair seating system is similar to piecing together a puzzle. The mystery lies in the fact that the sizes and shapes of the puzzle pieces change depending upon how the puzzle is viewed by the clinician. Assessment and selection of equipment components for patients who have sustained brain injury is a valuable learning experience for those involved with this aspect of the therapeutic program. This skill challenges the clinician to develop foresight by anticipating how the puzzle pieces fit together and how to integrate financial, physical, social, and cognitive variables in the scheme successfully. A clinician's skill in assessment for and selection of equipment components is vital to a comprehensive treatment program to lessen impairments and enhance functional outcomes for the individual who has sustained brain injury.

SUGGESTED READINGS

Bobath B: Adult Hemiplegia: Evaluation and Treatment. William Heinemann, London, 1978

Borello-France D, Burdett R, Gee Z: Modification of sitting posture of patients with hemiplegia using seat boards and backboards. Phys Ther 68:67, 1988

Carey JH, Burghart TP: Movement dysfunction following central nervous system lesions: a problem of neurologic or muscular impairment. Phys Ther 8:538, 1973

Duncan W: Tonic reflexes of the foot. J Bone Joint Surg 42A:859, 1960

Falk Bergen A, Presperin J, Tallman T: Positioning for Function. Valhalla Rehabilitation Publications, Ltd., Valhalla, NY, 1990

Fisher B: Effect of trunk control and alignment on limb function. J Head Trauma Rehabil 2:72, 1987

Fisher B, Yakura J: Movement analysis: a different perspective. Orthop Phys Ther Clin North Am 2:1, 1993

Hagen C, Malkmus D, Durham P: Levels of Cognitive Functioning in Rehabilitation of the Head Injured Adult: Comprehensive Physical Management. Rancho Los Amigos Medical Center, Downey, CA, 1979

Letts RM: Principles of Seating the Disabled. CRC Press, Boca Raton, FL, 1991

Peterson M, Adkins H: Measurement and redistribution of excessive pressures during wheelchair sitting. Phys Ther 62:990, 1982

7 | Orthotic Management of the Lower Extremity

Jan Utley
Cynthia Stone Thomas

Traumatic brain injury results in neuromuscular disturbances requiring lower extremity orthotics for the management of movement dysfunction in the foot and ankle. The purpose of an orthosis is to provide a stable base of support, promote postural control, and provide for more normal transitional movement strategies in function.

Examples of postural control factors and transitional movement strategies include sitting to standing, transfers from wheelchairs to various surfaces, getting into and out of a car, functional locomotion (including forward and backward progressions), sidestepping, turning, bending and reaching in function, and control in stepping up and down to a variety of surface heights. These strategies are basic to movement control in daily function. All of the aforementioned movement strategies require a stable base of support through the lower extremities, which can be aided by an orthotic device.

The primary purpose of an ankle-foot orthosis is to improve biomechanical alignment and provide more normal mobility and control in the lower extremity with weight bearing over the base of support. Selecting or constructing an orthosis requires an understanding of normal biomechanics in the foot and ankle. The proximal lower extremity and trunk must be analyzed in relation to foot and ankle control in functional movement. Specific problems with alignment and movement dysfunction in the client's foot must be assessed in weight-bearing and non-weight-bearing postures.

This chapter presents the rationale and guidelines for designing ankle-foot orthoses, including analysis of the structure and function of the normal and pathologic foot. Case studies will be presented demonstrating the use of a variety of orthoses utilized with head injured clients.

POSTURAL GROUNDING

Postural grounding (Thomas/Utley), a new concept to be considered in designing an orthosis for the foot and ankle, can be defined as the use of weight-bearing surfaces for spatial orientation and control of the body against gravity. The plantar surfaces of the feet, palmar surfaces of the hands, and ischial tuberosities of the pelvis are critical contact areas to permit the body (soma) to access and use somata-sensory information that contributes to skeletal muscle control in function. Although this discussion concentrates on the plantar surface of the foot in relation to lower extremity mobility, it is important to realize that utilization of these three surfaces develops in a parallel manner in infancy. Postural grounding occurs in normal infant development through the integration of plantar reflexes with weight bearing in movement from horizontal into vertical postures as righting and equilibrium develop. Normal infants seek information from the environment through their feet within the first 6 months of life. Exploration begins in the first 4 months, as the hands and feet come together in supine, and continues to be reinforced through environmental conditions created by baby furniture, supports, and handling. Parental handling also enhances the development of postural grounding as babies are held and bounced in standing and sitting. The plantar surfaces of the feet, palmar surfaces of the hands, and ischial tuberosities of the pelvis function as "kinesthetic eyes of the body" as they process information from and about the environment; in this way they assist with the development of normal righting and equilibrium responses. Throughout adult life these areas of weight-bearing contact with the supporting surface contribute to graded skeletal muscle coactivation in the extremities and the trunk. Movement over these surfaces also provides the individual with information about his or her position in relation to weight-bearing surfaces.

More complete plantar contact and distribution of weight-bearing pressures as the body moves over the foot require sufficient mobility in the foot and ankle. Appropriate plantar contact is a primary contributing factor for graded skeletal muscle activity up the kinetic chain in the lower extremity. The current and accepted definition of the term *kinetic chain* is the order of related muscle activity and timing of related muscle firing. One might relate this to synergistic organization. These events are also influenced by the starting postural alignment. When the feet, hands, and ischial tuberosities are not used, for whatever reason, other pats of the body may access somato-sensory feedback. This is often seen in individuals with poor head and trunk control. The head will seek a surface for weight bearing such as the surface of the bed or the backrest of a wheelchair. Individuals in wheelchairs with their feet on footrests are unable to access the necessary contact on the ground through the plantar surfaces of the feet. Depending upon the concentration of pressure through the bottom of the foot on the footrest, the foot may assume tonic postures of dorsiflexion or plantar flexion. The outcome of using other surfaces to gather somatic information might be the loss of the potential for automatic postural reactions involved in more normal weight bearing through the feet.

An ankle orthosis should encourage postural grounding by providing for mobility and control in the foot as the body moves over the base of support in function.

OVERVIEW OF STRUCTURAL ALIGNMENT AND FUNCTION IN THE NORMAL FOOT

Components of mobility and stability in the normal foot are determined by skeletal alignment and neuromuscular control of the articulations of the ankle and foot. In addition, proximal control throughout the lower extremity and trunk also influences alignment and control in the foot and ankle. Assessment of the following articulations in the ankle and foot are critical to the design and fabrication of an effective ankle-foot orthosis:

The ankle joint (talocrural)
The subtalar joint (talocalcaneal)
The midtarsal joint
   lateral (calcaneocuboid)
   medial (talonavicular)
The forefoot (cuneiforms, metatarsals, phalanges) (Fig. 7-1)

It is important to recognize that all of these articulations contribute to both stability and mobility components of function in the foot. There have been a number of biomechanical views of the structural alignment of the bones and joints of the foot. One view proposed by Paul Jordan in 1989 functionally divided the foot into lateral and medial columns. For purposes of this discussion, we use the following alignment: The lateral column (considered to be the more stable unit of the foot) includes the calcaneus, cuboid, second, and third cuneiforms, second through fifth metatarsals and phalanges. The medial (more mobile column) includes the talus, navicular, medial cuneiform first metatarsal and its phalanges (Steve Reischel, Rehabilitation Institute of Chicago, 1993). Normally, as the body moves over the foot in weight bearing, the medial column moves obliquely on the lateral column. Movement of the medial column downward toward the weight-bearing surface allows for more plantar conformation on the weight-bearing surface. Any movement of the medial column in an upward direction results in more stability in the foot. These components of function in the foot, combined with ankle range into dorsiflexion and plantar flexion must be considered in the design of the ankle-foot orthosis.

Tonic Reflexes of the Foot

In addition to structural components of the ankle and foot, it is imperative to recognize the importance of the development and integration of the tonic reflexes of the foot, first described by Duncan in 1960. There are four major

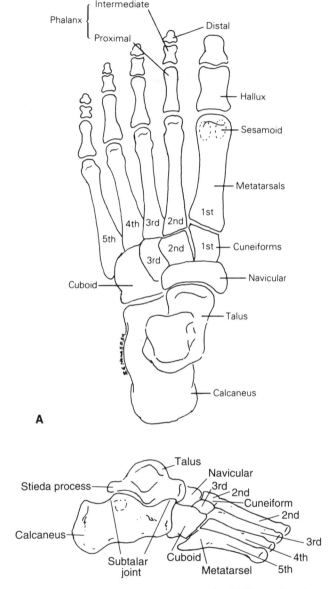

Fig. 7-1. Bones of the foot and ankle. (A) Dorsal. (B) Lateral. (From Subotnick A: Sports Medicine of the Lower Extremity. Churchill Livingstone, New York, 1989, p. 78, with permission.)

tonic reflexes of the foot: inversion, eversion, plantar flexion, and dorsiflexion responses. These reflexes, present at birth, affect the newborn's foot posturing. In the normal infant, with the development of weight bearing in the upright posture and ambulation, these reflexes become fully integrated.

In clients with traumatic brain injury the tonic reflex activity in the foot is a significant consideration in designing any orthosis. In addition to the use of an orthosis for more controlled biomechanical alignment of the foot, plantar inserts can be incorporated into the surface of the footplate. These build-ups can stimulate plantar reflexes that inhibit undesired patterns and encourage better plantar contact and muscle control in the stance and swing phases of gait.

Integration of the plantar reflexes results in the spread of the foot and conformation to weight-bearing surfaces. Therefore, we believe that the contours of the footplate should allow for changes in plantar contact as the body moves over the foot in weight bearing. There are a variety of options for plantar inserts, depending upon the specific biomechanical and tonic problems intrinsic to the foot as well as extrinsic factors. Medial inserts can be placed under the first metatarsal head, the navicular, or the plantar surfaces of the medial calcaneus. These inserts are effective for corrections in feet presenting with subtalar valgus or midtarsal pronation. If there is exaggerated varus in the hindfoot, midtarsal supination, or plantar flexion of the first ray, the footplate may require surface inserts under the fifth metatarsal head, the cuboid, or the lateral aspect of the plantar surface of the calcaneus. It is not necessary to use all of the points of stimulation described above, but one or two may be very effective, depending on the problems of dysfunction in the individual patient's foot.

GUIDELINES FOR DESIGNING ANKLE FOOT ORTHOSES

A number of guiding principle must be considered in designing any ankle-foot orthosis. A complete and accurate biomechanical evaluation of the patient's foot and ankle is essential. This includes assessment of available range of motion (ROM) in the following joints: the ankle, subtalar, medial and lateral midtarsal, first ray, and the remaining forefoot.

Assessing the foot neurobiologically is also important, including problems with hyperreflexia (such as stiffness and exaggerated tonic reflexes) and abnormal recruitment of skeletal muscle in the foot and ankle. Proximal control in the lower extremity and the trunk also affect foot and ankle function, and, therefore, must be included as part of the assessment.

Range of motion and skeletal muscle function should be analyzed in weight-bearing and non-weight-bearing strategies.

Before casting for fabrication of an orthosis, preparation of the foot and ankle may be necessary for obtaining desired alignment. This may involve mobilization if there are areas of stiffness in the foot and ankle. Trunk mobilization for better alignment in sitting or standing may also be required so that the foot and ankle may be casted for the orthosis in weight bearing.

Orthotics should be used as adjuncts in therapeutic intervention to help maintain alignment and control over the base of support for better carryover into function. The effectiveness of any orthosis depends upon the therapist's ability to help the patient achieve better control of movement in function.

Over time, as the patient improves, an orthosis should be modified. These modifications are generally characterized by a gradual withdrawal of control and should be made on the average every 8 to 12 months. Some examples in head-injured patients include moving from more rigid to more flexible materials or progressing from more support to less support. Another example might be changing from a hinged below ankle-foot orthosis to a dorsal ankle-foot orthosis, and later possibly a supra malleolar or Utley Foot Orthosis (UFO). Eventually, some patients will progress to a level of control requiring the use of a simple plantar insert. Each succeeding orthosis then allows for more access to ROM and better muscle control in the ankle and foot.

External modifications of shoes such as buttresses, plantar wedging on the sole of the shoe, modified strapping and tying configurations, as well as the type of shoe to be worn with the orthosis are important factors. Generally, it is only necessary to purchase a shoe one-half to one size larger with the orthoses discussed in this chapter. Shoes that are more than one size larger tend to interfere with more normal somato-sensory feedback through the foot and lower extremity.

The design of an orthosis should correct and improve abnormal biomechanical alignment in the foot and ankle and encourage more normal muscle activation in function. Collaboration of the therapist and the orthotist is critical in the design, casting, and fitting of orthoses.

ANKLE AND FOOT MOBILIZATION

The mobilization techniques presented here developed over the past 12 years and originated with the two authors. They have been further modified during the past 3 years by Robert Landel, Steve Reischel, and Beth Fisher. The modifications have been determined by the specific neuromuscular problems involved with joint stiffness in neurologically impaired patients.

Tibiotalar Mobilization

Tibio-talar mobilization involves talar glides posteriorly on the tibia and fibula. The following two figures demonstrate the hand placements for gliding the talus posteriorly on the tibia for increased ankle range and dorsiflexion. If possible, align the hindfoot in subtalar neutral and maintain this alignment as the following pressures are applied.

The pressures on the plantar surface are distraction along the longitudinal axis of the foot followed by pressure toward dorsiflexion. The dorsal pressure is applied simultaneously with the pressure into dorsiflexion and is directed backward toward the heel. Movement of the tibia in a backward displacement is prevented by the plantar distraction and by stabilizing the patient's knee with the therapist's shoulder or head (Fig. 7-2).*

Subtalar Mobilization

Subtalar joint mobilization to increase range into valgus is achieved through the application of pressure on the calcaneus in an oblique direction from lateral to medial. Figure 7-3 demonstrates the hand placements for applying this pressure. The thumbs overlap on the lateral aspect of the calcaneus and pressure is applied with the top thumb through the thumb directly on the hindfoot. This provides a cushion effect as this pressure is sometimes noxious. The navicular must be stabilized medially as the pressure is applied to the calcaneus to provide a point of stability on which to move the hindfoot into valgus. The knee must also be stabilized medially to prevent hip adduction. The therapist can accomplish this by stabilizing with the chin on the medial aspect of the knee.

Midtarsal Mobilization

Midtarsal joint mobilization involves movement of the navicular medially and downward on the talus. The hand placements and pressures are demonstrated in Figure 7-4. The hindfoot is held in neutral as pressure is applied across the navicular in an oblique direction from lateral to medial. To provide more comfort, use the thenar eminence to apply this pressure across the navicular.

First Ray Mobilization

Mobilization of the first ray involves pressure against the medial cuneiform and proximal aspect of the first metatarsal in an oblique medial direction. The hindfoot is stabilized in neutral with the index finger on the process of the navicular to prevent pronation in the midtarsal joint. Pressure on the dorsum is across the medial cuneiform and the first metatarsal joint. Pressure on the dorsum is across the medial cuneiform and the first metatarsal in an oblique direction from lateral to medial. For a cushioning effect, the pressure is applied through the thenar eminence (Figs. 7-5 and 7-6).

---

* All photographs in this chapter copyright Kari Alberthal, Southern Methodist University, Dallas, TX, 1993.

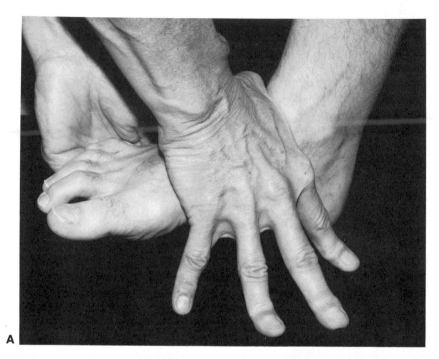

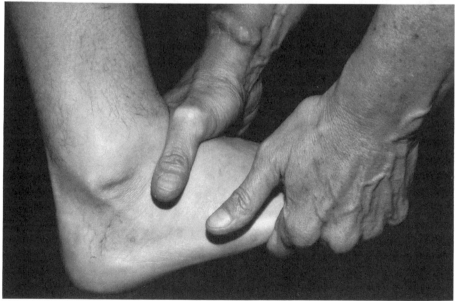

Fig. 7-2.   (A&B) Tibiotalar mobilization.

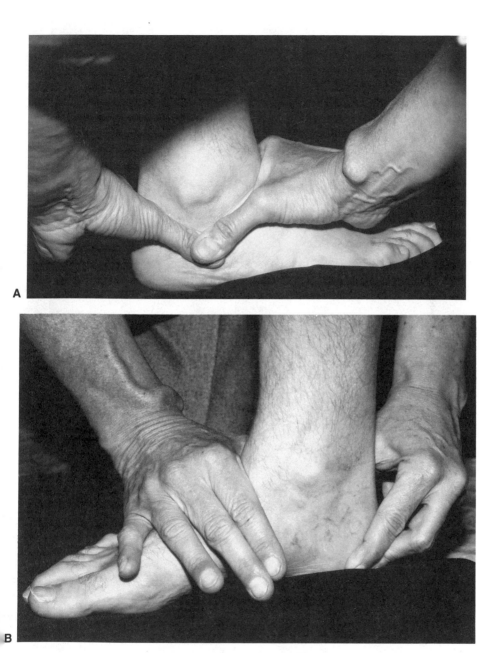

Fig. 7-3.   (A&B) Subtalar joint mobilization.

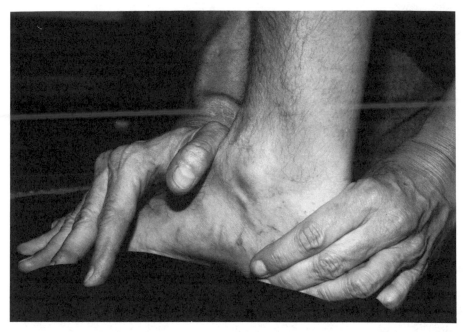

Fig. 7-4. Midtarsal joint mobilization.

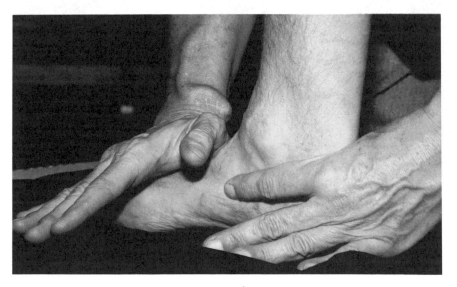

Fig. 7-5. Mobilization of the first ray.

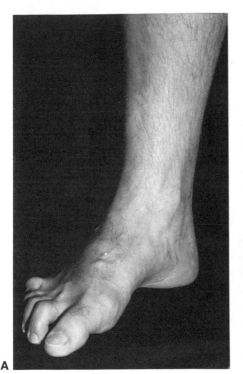
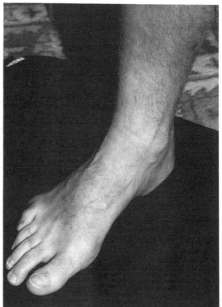

A   B

Fig. 7-6. (A&B) Demonstration of the effectiveness of the mobilization of the first ray on a client whose ankle was stiff with hindfoot and midfoot supination and had an elevated first ray.

CASE STUDIES

The following case studies demonstrate a range of problems in the foot and ankle from minimal to severe abnormal alignments and movement dysfunction. Each case study includes an assessment of problems and the rationale for the types of ankle-foot orthoses used to resolve them and to promote improved alignment and muscle control.

Case 1

The patient sustained a head injury in an automobile accident in November 1983. Initially, he required a tracheotomy and was comatose for 3 months.

He was referred for treatment in January 1985 with primary involvement on the left side of the body and minimal problems in the right lower extremity. The left foot was stiff in plantar flexion with strong "clawing" of the toes. The left lower extremity was assessed in weight-bearing activities such as transfers, sitting to standing, and gait. The primary problems observed and felt in the foot and ankle were stiffness and resistance to tibial movement forward over the talus (posterior talar glide). The subtalar joint was stiff and remained in excessive varus during weight bearing. There was also stiffness in the medial component of the midtarsal joint. The tibiotalar and subtalar immobility resulted in resistance to movement of the medial column down toward the weight-bearing surface as he attempted to load the left leg. The toe "clawing" could have been his attempt to seek contact with the ground medially. This patient could not shift weight onto the left lower extremity and therefore maintained his body mass primarily over the right side, causing classic compensatory "overuse" syndrome. Non-weight-bearing assessment of ROM confirmed all of the findings noted in weight-bearing functions.

Therapist intervention included manual mobilization of the areas of stiffness in the left ankle and foot. Mobilization techniques were followed immediately with use of graded ROM in weight-bearing activities such as transitional movements of sitting to standing and functional locomotion.

To help maintain the ROM achieved through mobilization and weight-bearing activities, a fiberglass "strip cast" night boot was used to control the ankle, subtalar joint, and midtarsal joint. Toe spreaders were fabricated bilaterally to control excessive toe flexion.

Mobilization techniques were also carried out before casting to prepare for the orthosis. The foot and ankle were cast in sitting with the foot in weight bearing. The alignment maintained in the casting procedure was 5° of dorsiflexion, with slight valgus in the subtalar joint. The toe spreader was worn on the foot during the casting procedure to inhibit the toe "clawing" and maintain the desired alignment throughout the foot. The orthosis, a modification of the UFO was designed to control the hindfoot at initial contact in a slight valgus alignment. This helps to bring the medial column down and provide for movement of the tibia forward over the foot as the lower extremity loads in walking. The upright and heel cup were constructed of $\frac{5}{32}$ inch polypropylene. The footplate was extended the length of the foot with a thin, more flexible piece of polyethylene plastic to provide for more flexibility in the forefoot and the metatarsal phalangeal joints toward terminal stance. A Gaffney joint was used medially to allow for full range in dorsiflexion and plantar flexion of the ankle. The buildup areas on the orthosis were of expanded polyethylene soft density foam. Velstretch velcro was used for strapping (except for the strap across the dorsum of the toes, which was sling webbing). The toe spreader was applied to the footplate as the client preferred it for convenience.

The use of more flexible materials and incorporation of a flat footplate (including the medial arch) in the design of this orthosis allows for full functional range in dorsiflexion and plantar flexion from initial contact, through midstance, to terminal stance in forward step progressions. It also stimulates plantar receptors laterally on the foot to help with movement toward pronation as the lower extremity loads in weight bearing. This is accomplished by building in a wedged surface on the lateral side of the footplate. The size of this wedging should be within a range of $\frac{1}{8}''$ to $\frac{1}{4}''$ on most clients. Excessive wedging will increase pressure on the lateral border of the foot and will have the opposite effect of inhibiting pronation. The medial configuration promotes medial/lateral stability in the ankle and hindfoot. These mobility and stability factors can be observed in the transition from sitting to standing. The differences are demonstrated in Figures 7-7 to 7-10.

Overall, this type of orthosis gave this patient the potential for increased activity. including the possibility of learning to run and ride a bicycle again. He had a vested interest in physical activity and sports as he was training for the Olympic Decathlon at the time of his injury.

Case 2

The patient was 21 years old when she sustained a head injury in an automobile accident in 1988. She was initially in a coma and on life support systems.

The initial condition of the foot and ankle resulted in severe equinovarus. Stiffness and plantar flexion, subtalar varus, with midfoot and forefoot supination/adduction made it impossible to bear weight on the left lower extremity. Bilateral heel cord releases were performed, which resolved the problems in the right foot, but the left foot remained supinated and inverted with a plantar flexed first ray. The patient could not bring the heel into contact with the ground when attempting weight bearing on the left lower extremity. Initially, a rigid ankle foot orthosis (traditional design with no access to ankle range and a rigid footplate with a high medial

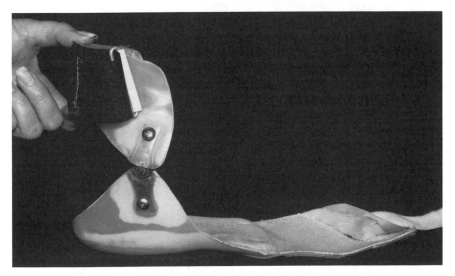

Fig. 7-7.   Medial view of hinged UFO.

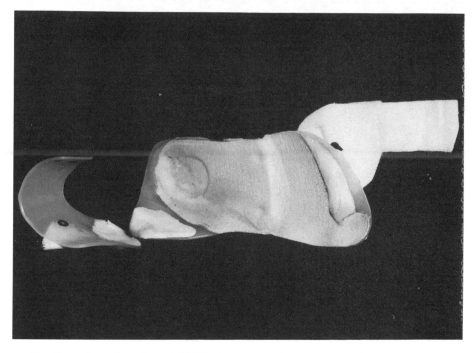

Fig. 7-8.   Superior view of UFO showing surface of foot plate with toe crest.

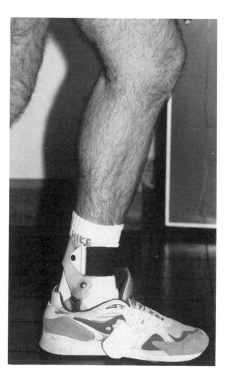

Fig. 7-9. Demonstration of client stepping forward showing allowance for range into dorsiflexion.

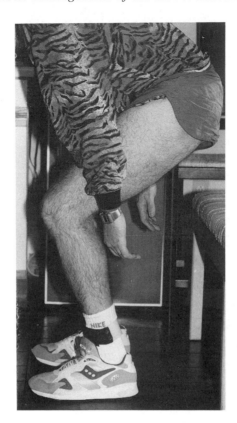

Fig. 7-10. Transitional movement from sitting to standing while wearing UFO.

longitudinal arch) was used. With this design it was still not possible to seat the hindfoot and achieve any weight bearing through the heel in standing or sitting.

In 1991 when we first saw and began working with this patient, she was confined to a wheelchair and not able to walk or even sit unsupported on a surface. Her foot was very stiff and required extensive mobilization to prepare for a new orthosis. The design of the orthotic device was a modification of the Dorsal Ankle Foot Orthosis (Nancy Hilton, P.T.). This type of orthosis came about through the collaborative efforts of Nicky Schmidt, P.T., and Deborah Merrit (M&R Prosthetics, New Orleans, LA). The material used for the orthotic was polyethylene. The footplate was rigid and the material was pulled very thin over the dorsum of the foot. The contour of the heel cup remained in approximately 5° of varus (the range achieved through mobilization of the foot). There was a slight buildup in the peroneal arch and under the fifth metatarsal head. A toe crest under the lateral four toes helped to inhibit severe toe clawing. In addition to this build-up on the footplate, a "toe-spreader" had to be added to control exaggerated flexion of the toes. The pelite on the bottom of the orthosis is wedged laterally $\frac{1}{4}''$ to facilitate more pronation in the foot as the tibia moves forward in weight bearing (Figs. 7-11 to 7-17).

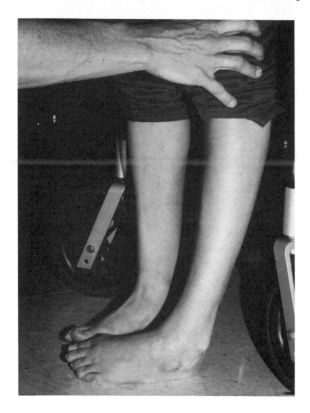

Fig. 7-11. Client coming to standing without orthosis.

The client has improved significantly in her functional skills. She now walks with assistance and can independently care for herself in toileting and in general bathroom functions. She can also stand at counter surfaces in the kitchen without assistance and can transfer independently. In all of these and other weight-bearing functions she has ground contact from the heel through the forefoot when wearing the orthosis. She will soon be evaluated for a new, more flexible orthosis because of increased mobility in the subtalar joint and the midtarsal articulation. This improvement has been achieved through continued foot mobilization and increased weight bearing in function.

Case 3

In April 1985 this 15-year-old patient sustained a head injury in an automobile accident. He was on life support systems for 5 days and comatose to semicomatose for 6 months. He was discharged to his home in October 1985, totally dependent but able to be propped and supported in a reclining wheelchair. He had no active head or trunk control and was referred for treatment in 1986.

The client presented with severe truncal stiffness characterized by

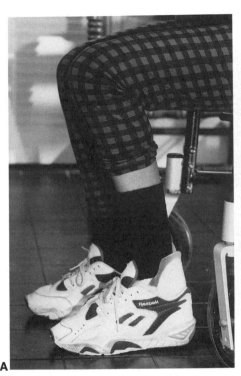
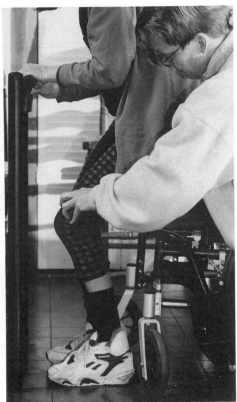

A   B

Fig. 7-12. (A&B) Transition from sitting to standing demonstrating improved alignment and mobility in foot and ankle. The patient's body can now move forward over her feet for better balance and control.

lateral flexion to the left and excessive posterior rotation of the pelvis on the femur. The cervical spine was rotated with the face turned to the left. The upper extremities were held stiffly in an alignment of shoulder abduction and hyperextension with elbow, wrist, and finger flexion. Although his hands were fisted bilaterally, he had some ability to open and close the left hand with the wrist in flexion. Both lower extremities were stiff in extension at all joints. Both feet and ankles were postured in plantar flexion, hindfoot varus, midtarsal pronation, and plantar flexion of the first ray with forefoot adduction. The toes were also stiffly flexed. No active movement was present in the lower extremities with the exception of slight movement in the left knee.

Following mobilization of the trunk and bilateral foot mobilization, the pelvis lacked 20° reaching neutral alignment (90°), and the feet could be maintained on the floor with input from the therapist. The left ankle was in 15° plantar flexion and the right ankle in 25°. The first ray was in

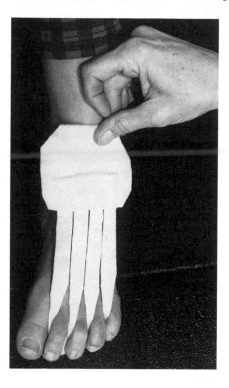

Fig. 7-13. Dorsal view of toe spreader.

contact with the floor; however, the midtarsal joint was still supinated and the subtalar joint was in varus. The right foot was more severely deformed than the left. It was not possible to move the body center of mass over the feet in sitting. In sitting to standing and in standing, the therapist had to maintain trunk extension. The patient could weight bear on the left foot, but only with the alignment described above. The right lower extremity was rotated back at the pelvis with knee hyperextension, ankle plantar

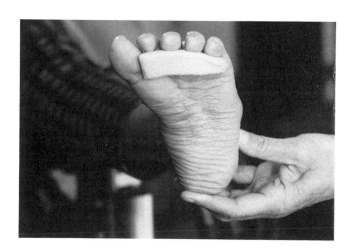

Fig. 7-14. Plantar view of toe spreader.

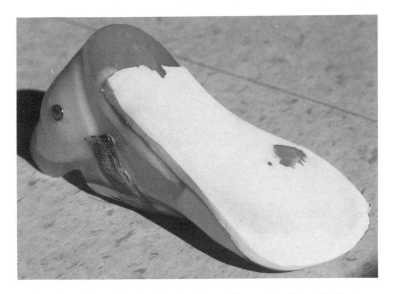

Fig. 7-15.   Plantar surface of orthosis showing pelite wedge laterally for increased pronation in weight bearing.

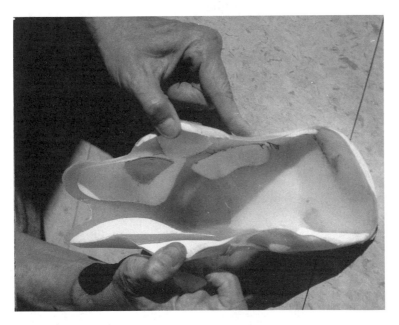

Fig. 7-16.   Thinned dorsal aspect of orthosis pulled to show lateral build-up for stimulation of pronation/eversion through the foot in weight bearing.

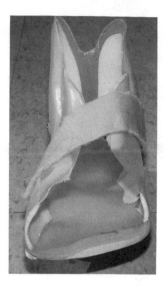

Fig. 7-17. Front view of dorsal ankle-foot orthosis showing single strap from lateral to medial to help maintain midtarsal pronation. The toe crest and lateral pelite wedge effect are visible as orthosis sits on weight-bearing surface.

flexion, and supination in the foot. Standing required the assistance of two people. Assessment of the tonic reflexes revealed hyperreflexive inversion in the forefoot, midfoot, and hindfoot. There was a very strong plantar flexion response with severe toe grasp. The right foot presented with tonic reflexes. There was no response to facilitation of the dorsiflexion or eversion reflexes in either foot.

Therapist intervention included the use of inhibitive "strip casts" with bilateral toe spreaders. The casts consisted of a footplate, a fiberglass slipper cast, a fiberglass posterior shell, and an anterior shell that could be removed for bathing and skin care. The footplate was designed to stimulate pronation and eversion through buildups under the peroneal arch and fifth metatarsal head bilaterally. The toe spreaders were used to inhibit exaggerated toe grasp. A two-inch wide velcro strap was added across the dorsum of the toes to help in maintaining them in extension on the footplate. All of the casting was performed with the client seated with the feet in weight bearing. The slipper cast had no medial arch and controlled the foot intrinsically. The posterior and anterior shell was designed to control dorsiflexion/plantar flexion factors. The slipper cast was modified twice as the foot improved and neutral alignment was obtained. The posterior shell was modified every month as increased range into dorsiflexion was achieved. The client remained in "strip casts" for nine months before he could be progressed into jointed orthoses (Figs. 7-18 to 7-23).

The first pair of jointed ankle-foot orthoses were cast with the client seated with the feet in weight bearing. Before casting, his trunk was mobilized to improve the alignment in sitting. Subtalar neutral was obtained in the casting procedure. The footplate is a flat surface (no medial arch) with a built-in toe crest. The orthosis was constructed of $\frac{5}{32}$ polypropylene with bilateral stainless steel popsicle hinges The upright molded cuff stopped

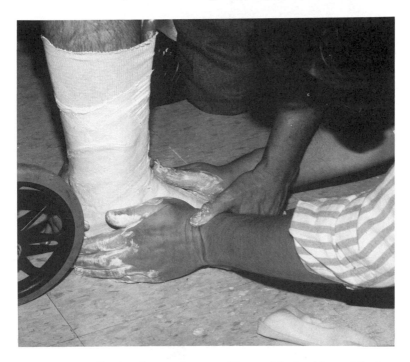

Fig. 7-18.   Casting for resultant positive mold of ankle and foot.

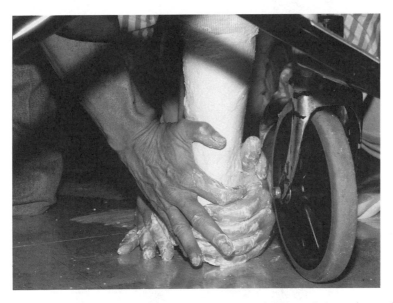

Fig. 7-19.   Posterior view of casting procedure. The orthotist and therapist are holding the joint in the desired alignment.

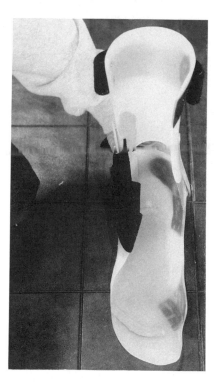

Fig. 7-20. Superior view showing foot plate with no medial arch, slight hindfoot valgus, and the toe crest.

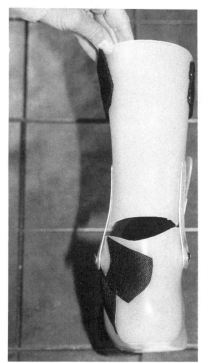

Fig. 7-21. Posterior view of orthosis showing alignment of hindfoot in slight valgus.

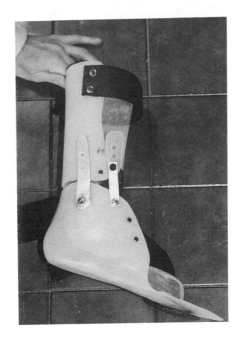

Fig. 7-22. Lateral view of orthosis showing popsicle hinge and device for adjustment to allow for more or less pronation depending upon whether client is sitting, in weight bearing, or walking. (There is less access to pronation during gait because of stiffness and hyperreflexia into plantar flexion).

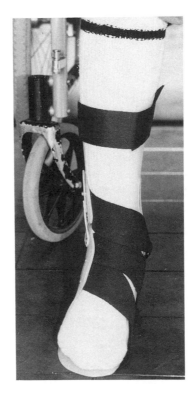

Fig. 7-23. Client is wearing the orthosis while weight bearing through lower extremities in sitting.

below the gastrocnemius muscle belly. The popsicle hinge allowed for dorsiflexion and approximately 8° of plantar flexion. A small lateral device can be adjusted to maintain a neutral ankle or permit some plantar flexion, depending on whether the client remains seated or is on his feet standing and walking. The strapping configuration is designed to pull from lateral to medial to enhance foot pronation.

ACKNOWLEDGMENT

All photographs in this chapter are by Kari Alberthal, Southern Methodist University, Dallas, Texas.

SUGGESTED READINGS

Donatelli R, Walker R: Lower quarter evaluation: structural relationships and interdependence. In Donatelli R, Wooden MJ (eds): Orthopaedic Physical Therapy. 2nd Ed. Churchill Livingstone, New York, 1994

Donatelli R: Biomechanics of the Foot and Ankle. FA Davis, Philadelphia, 1992

Horak FB, Shumway-Cook A: New Perspective on Balance and Coordination: Neurophysiological Basis for Evaluation and Treatment. Instructional Syllabus

Hylton N: Postural and functional impact of dynamic AFOs and FOs in a pediatric population. J Prosthetics Orthotics 2:40, 1986

Kottke FJ, et al: Rationale for prolonged stretching for correction of shortened connective issue. Arch Phys Med Rehabil 6:345, 1966

Landel R, Fisher B: Musculoskeletal considerations in the neurologically impaired patient. Orthopaedic Physical Therapy Clinics of North America, WB Saunders, March 1993

Lehneis HR: New concepts in lower extremity orthotics. Med Clin North Am 53: 585, 1969

Montgomery J: Orthotic management of the lower limb in head-injured adults. J of Head Trauma Rehabilitation 2:57, 1987

Observational Gait Analysis: 1993. Rancho Los Amigos Research and Education Institute, Inc., Downey, CA

Perry J: Gait Analysis: Normal and Pathological Function. Slack Inc., Thorofare, NJ, 1992

Reischl S, Fisher M: Orthopaedic Management of the Neurological Foot and Ankle. Lab Manual, Rehabilitation Institute of Chicago, Nov 1993

Shamp J: Neurophysiological ankle foot orthosis. Clinical Prosthetics and Orthotics 10:15, 1986

8 | Reconstructive Surgery for Residual Lower Extremity Deformities

Douglas E. Garland

Definitive surgical procedures are not performed until one and one-half years have elapsed after the initial head injury.[1] Further motor recovery is minimal after this time. Surgery adds another dimension to the rehabilitation process and may be a useful modality in gaining independence. Surgery should be considered a form of rehabilitation, since it aids in restoring normalcy and may render devices unnecessary.

The selection of a surgical procedure depends upon observation during performance, not at the bedside. Diagnostic procaine nerve blocks further refine the selection of tendon lengthening, release, and/or transfer preoperatively for the surgeon. Nerve blocks give the patient, family, and therapist an insight to the predicted surgical outcome. Kinesiologic electromyography (i.e., a gait laboratory or dynamic electromyographs) offer precise insight into the selective process of proper tendon release, lengthening, or transfer when available.

NONFUNCTIONAL SURGERY

The main reasons for nonfunctional surgery are to improve hygiene, and relieve pain, and, occasionally, to assist in activities of daily living. These surgeries consist mainly in the release of contractures. It may be necessary to perform surgery in the low-level patient less than $1\frac{1}{2}$ years after the initial insult if myostatic contractures are present. Diagnostic nerve blocks and dynamic electromyography are usually not indicated. In some instances, patients who require nonfunctional releases have been neglected early and develop contractures even though some functional potential may exist.[2]

Hip

Flexion Contracture

Surgical indications: pain, hygiene, ease nursing care
Surgery: anterior hip release
Postoperative management: stretching exercises and proning

This deformity occurs in the neglected patient and the patient with severe neurologic compromise, especially the quadriparetic. Surgery consists of a standard anterior approach to the hip, releasing the hip flexor muscles. The anterior incision should avoid the anterior superior iliac spine so that proning may be utilized postoperatively without causing wound compromise. Adduction contractures are usually present, although these are mild in comparison to the primary adduction deformity (Fig. 8-1). Surgery for this combined deformity consists of a percutaneous adductor release prior to the formal anterior release of the hip flexors.

Adduction Contracture

Surgical indications: pain, hygiene, ease nursing care
Surgery: adductor muscle release and anterior obturator neurectomy
Postoperative management: passive stretching exercises, abduction splint

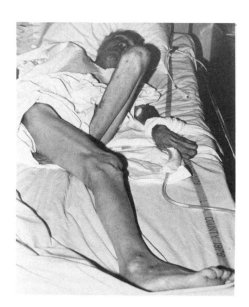

Fig. 8-1. This patient presents two hip deformities. The left hip has a "primary" hip flexion deformity with a mild adductor contracture. Corrective surgery would consist of percutaneous adductor release and an anterior hip release. A left knee release is also indicated. The right hip displays a "primary" adduction contracture with a mild hip flexion deformity. Corrective surgery would consist of an adductor muscle release, an anterior obturator neurectomy, and an iliopsoas muscle release.

A standard medial approach to the adductor muscles is performed, releasing the adductor longus, adductor brevis and gracilis muscles from their origin. The anterior obturator nerve is sectioned. A complete obturator neurectomy and release of the adductor magnus muscle may lead to an abduction deformity. The adduction contracture is often associated with a mild flexion deformity which is not as severe as the primary hip flexion deformity previously mentioned (Fig. 8-1). When the mild hip flexion deformity is present, the iliopsoas tendon is released through the same incision as the adductor muscle release.

Knee

Flexion Contracture

Surgical indications: pain, hygiene, ease nursing care
Surgery: hamstring muscle release
Postoperative management: serial casting or dropout casts followed by anterior-posterior splinting, passive stretching

Knee flexion contractures are usually associated with hip flexion deformities. As the hip flexion contracture develops, the knee assumes a flexed position and develops a contracture conversely. Release of all the hamstring muscles is performed through midlateral and medial incisions or through a midposterior knee incision. The contracture is usually not fully corrected at surgery. Capsular releases of the knee are rarely indicated. Once the muscles are released and the knee is extended, the neurovascular structures become taut preventing further extension. This negates any benefits of capsular releases. Serial long-leg casts or dropout casts aid in correcting the remaining contracture. If hip and knee contractures are released at the same surgery, the residual hip and knee deformities may be corrected after surgery as necessary. As the patient is positioned prone, a dropout cast of the leg aids in gaining extension of the knee (Fig. 8-2).

FUNCTIONAL SURGERY

Functional surgery is indicated to aid in controlling a deformity within an orthotic device, to eliminate an orthotic device, or to improve function. Methods in predicting surgical outcome are the diagnostic procaine nerve blocks and dynamic electromyography. Spastic muscles do not change phase after transfer, which sometimes occurs in normal transferred muscles.[3] Therefore, a spastic swing-phase muscle must not be transferred to substitute for a stance-phase muscle. This spastic transferred muscle will not convert to stance activity. Electromyography assists in the selection of a proper tendon transfer.

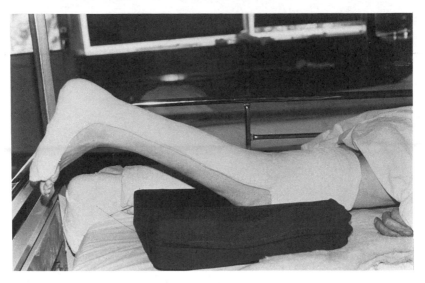

Fig. 8-2.   A dropout cast of the leg. While the patient is being proned the anterior hip contracture is stretched. Gravity aids in gaining extension of the knee. The posterior shell of the tibial portion of the cast prevents knee flexion while the patient is supine.

Hip

Hypertonic Hip Extensors

Surgical indication: inadequate hip flexion during gait
Surgery: proximal hamstring recession (release)
Postoperative management: passive hamstring stretching and gait training

This deformity is uncommon. It results from residual extensor patterning and is frequently associated with a stiff-legged gait of the knee and an equinus posturing of the ankle. The gait deformity may be masked by hypermobility of the lumbar spine. The patient may not be able to flex his hip when standing erect but has near full flexion when supine. Hamstring tightness is usually present. The hamstrings are released from their origin and allowed to slide distally. Surgery allows increased hip motion, cadence and stride length (Fig. 8-3).

Hypertonic Hip Adductors

Surgical indication: scissoring during ambulation
Surgery: selective release of the adductor muscles
Postoperative management: gait training

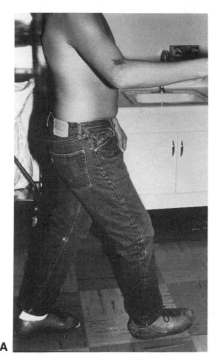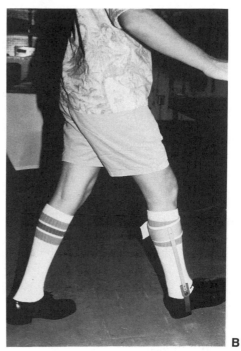

A   B

Fig. 8-3. **(A)** Hypertonic hip extensors. The patient has decreased stride length. **(B)** The patient has undergone a proximal hamstring recession. Extensor patterning is decreased and the patient now has increased stride length.

As opposed to the adductor release of nonfunctional surgery, this surgery is performed in the ambulatory patient. Hip motion is full, with no evidence of contracture. A procaine obturator nerve block aids in predicting ambulatory gains. A percutaneous release of the adductor muscles is usually performed. This is in contradistinction to the nonfunctional surgery, wherein all adductor muscles (except the adductor magnus muscle) are released and the anterior obturator nerve is excised. A percutaneous tenotomy sufficiently weakens the adductors, preventing the dynamic deformity but allowing adequate strength for gait. If available, a gait analysis electromyography is an excellent method of identifying the abnormally spastic muscle or muscles. A selective release of the offending muscle is then performed.

Knee

Hypertonic Quadriceps

Surgical indication: stiff-legged gait
Surgery: selective quadriceps release
Postoperative management: gait training

This is one of the more common and classic deformities of hemiplegia. Presently, this procedure is only performed if preoperative dynamic electromyographs are available.[4] Although this deformity is common, most patients fail to meet strict abnormal electromyographic criteria for surgical release. Consequently, few patients undergo this procedure. The spastic quadriceps muscles prevent knee flexion when they are active at "heel-off" on the involved extremity. A selective release above the knee of the vastus intermedius and the rectus femoris muscles, singly or in combination, is performed when they are deemed electromyographically out of phase. A release of the vastus medialis or lateralis muscles is not undertaken due to possible dislocation of the patella postoperatively.

Hypertonic Hamstrings

Surgical indication: crouched gait
Surgery: selective hamstring release
Postoperative management: gait training

In the nonfunctional surgery, all hamstrings are released. Dynamic electromyographs identify the hyperactive hamstring muscles. The hamstrings that are out of phase or active during midstance are surgically released (Fig. 8-4). If dynamic electromyographs are not available, identification by palpation of the spastic hamstrings during gait or by the palpated tight hamstring at surgery with subsequent release may offer less crouching with improved gait.

Ankle

Equinus

Surgical indications: contracture, orthotic containment, brace-free ambulation
Surgery: tendo-Achilles lengthening
Postoperative management: short leg walking cast for 6 weeks followed by an ankle-foot-orthosis (AFO) for 6 weeks

Equinus is the most common deformity of the hemiplegic lower extremity. Surgery is very predictable and successful; however, lengthening the tendon-Achilles the precise amount is often difficult. A mildly weakened calf muscle or persistent mildly overactive muscles are as common as near normal calf strength after lengthening. Many patients become brace-free after surgery. A smaller number of patients are operated upon to allow containment of the ankle in an orthosis. A diagnostic posterior tibialis nerve block posteriorly at the knee aids in predicting brace-free ambulation and in differentiating between spastic and weak calf muscles. Proprioception of the foot should be present before brace-free ambulation can be positively predicted. The percutaneous hemisec-

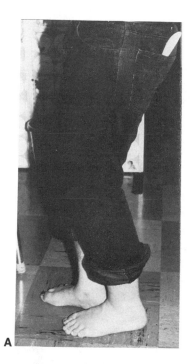

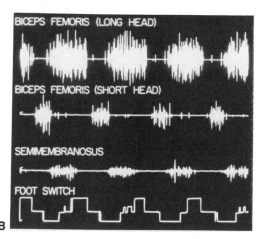

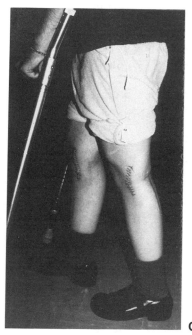

Fig. 8-4. (**A**) The patient presents with a crouched gait, which is secondary to hamstring muscles acting at midstance. (**B**) Dynamic electromyograph of the patient. The semi-membranosus and long biceps femoris muscles are out of phase and abnormally active at the midstance phase of normal gait. The baseline of the "footswitch" is the swing phase of gait. (**C**) The same patient postoperatively. Release of the semimembranosus and long biceps femoris muscles was performed.

tion of the heel cord lengthening of Hoke is preferred and may be performed under local anesthesia if necessary.[5-7] Occasionally, only the gastrocnemius muscle is hyperactive, as shown by gait electromyography. In this instance, a gastrocnemius muscle resection may be performed. The toes often curl or remain in a plantar flexed position when the ankle assumes a neutral attitude. Consequently, the common toe flexors are concomitantly released when a heel cord lengthening is performed. Gait training commences when pain and swelling subside in the short leg walking cast.

Heel

Heel Varus

Surgical indications: pain, orthotic containment, brace-free ambulation
Surgery: lengthening of posterior tibialis muscle
Postoperative management: short leg walking cast for 6 weeks

This deformity represents isolated ankle or heel varus and not varus of the hindfoot, which is frequently associated with varus of the forefoot. In this instance, minimal forefoot varus is present with significant varus at the heel (Fig. 8-5). The hyperactive posterior tibialis muscle is confirmed by a procaine posterior tibialis nerve block at the knee. If the deformity persists after the nerve block, the deformity is secondary to the anterior tibialis muscle. The anterior tibialis muscle causes forefoot varus with consequent heel varus. The posterior tibial tendon may be lengthened proximal or distal to the medial malleolus. Electromyographic evidence demonstrates that this muscle is frequently inactive in acquired spasticity; in only certain specific instances, when documented by dynamic electromyography or nerve block, should lengthening of the posterior tibialis muscles be undertaken.[8,9] Gait training begins when pain and swelling have subsided after surgery.

Forefoot

Forefoot Varus

Surgical indications: pain, orthotic containment, brace-free ambulation
Surgery: split anterior tibial tendon transfer (SPLATT)
Postoperative management: short leg walking cast for 6 weeks, AFO during the day and posterior splint at night for 4 months.

This is not common as an isolated deformity but is usually associated with spastic calf muscles.[5-7] Patients frequently discard their orthosis if this is an isolated deformity even though it controls the deformity adequately. If this

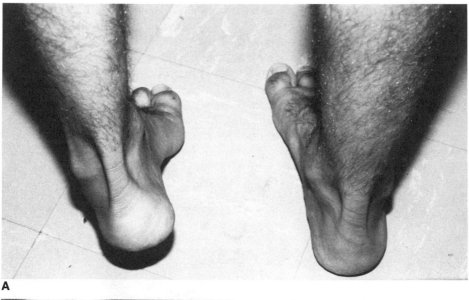

A

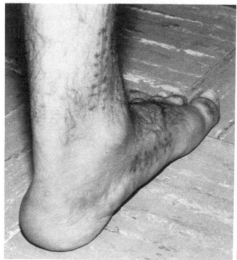

B

Fig. 8-5. (A) Significant heel varus without corresponding forefoot varus. (B) The posterior tibialis muscle has been lengthened at the ankle.

deformity is isolated, the patient will predictably have a balanced forefoot and become brace-free postoperatively.

Planovalgus Foot

Surgical indication: pain in the arch of the foot

Surgery: muscle transfer to the arch of the foot (and also a tendo-Achilles lengthening)

Postoperative management: short leg walking cast for 6 weeks, an ankle-foot orthosis (AFO) with longitudinal arch support for 3 to 4 months

These patients display a predisposition to flat feet, as can be detected on the contralateral extremity (Fig. 8-6). The posterior tibialis muscle is almost always inactive on the dynamic electromyogram; consequently the support to the arch of the foot is diminished. The third common finding is an overactive calf muscle, which adds to the stress and eventual breakdown at the mid arch of the foot during the stance phase of gait. Surgery usually involves heel cord lengthening in conjunction with transfer of a posterior or stance-phase muscle anteriorly. The transferred muscle may be routed through the interosseous membrane or subcutaneously around the fibula and sutured into the normal insertion of the posterior tibialis muscle on the tarsal navicular bone. An in-phase transfer is performed, usually a toe flexor or peroneus longus muscle, which now supports the arch during the stance phase of gait. A permanent longitudinal arch support may be necessary.

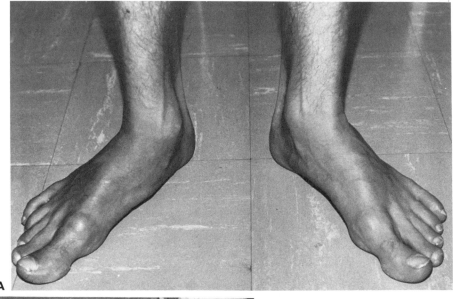

A

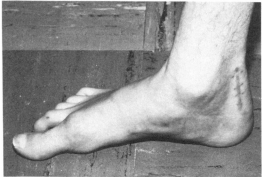

Fig. 8-6. (A) A planovalgus foot is present on the left. A predisposition to this deformity is noted by the pes planus (flat foot) deformity on the right. (B) A heel cord lengthening and transfer of the peroneus longus muscle anteriorly has been performed.

B

Cavus

Surgical indication: foot containment in shoes, pain
Surgery: plantar fascia release
Postoperative management: serial short leg casts may be necessary to correct
   the deformity

This deformity is uncommon (Fig. 8-7A). The equinus occurs in the forefoot and not the heel. Donning and wearing footwear may be difficult and cause pain. In long-standing deformities, excision of the plantar fascia may be necessary (Fig. 8-7B).

Forefoot, Heel, and Ankle Varus

Surgical indication: foot containment in shoes
Surgery: posteriomedial release of the ankle, lengthening of posterior tibialis
   muscle, plantar fascia release
Postoperative management: serial casts for 6 weeks

This deformity is rare (Fig. 8-8). It is most commonly observed in the severely involved patient but does not cause clinical problems in the low-level patient. However, should the patient demonstrate considerable neurologic improvement, this deformity may prevent the wearing of shoes.

Toes

Curling

Surgical indication: pain
Surgery: release of the flexor hallucis longus and flexor digitorum communis
   tendons
Postoperative management: none

True toe curling represents flexion of both the proximal and distal interphalangeal joints. If all the toes demonstrate curling, a release of the common toe flexor and hallus longus tendons is performed in the arch of the foot. If only one or two toes are curling, the long toe flexors are released at each individual toe. This procedure is routinely performed with tendo-Achilles lengthening. Even though toe curling may not be present preoperatively, the deformity commonly becomes evident once the ankle attains a neutral position.

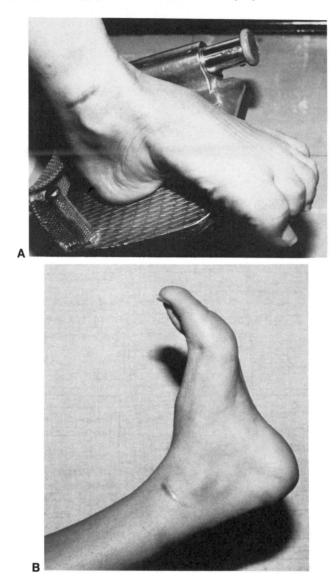

Fig. 8-7. (A) Forefoot equinus. Donning shoes was difficult, as was maintaining the foot in the shoe. (B) A plantar fascia release has been performed (and also toe flexor releases). No casting was necessary for this patient.

Flexion of the Proximal Interphalangeal Joint (with Hyperextension of the Distal Interphalangeal Joint)

Surgical indication: pain
Surgery: release of short toe flexor tendons
Postoperative management: none

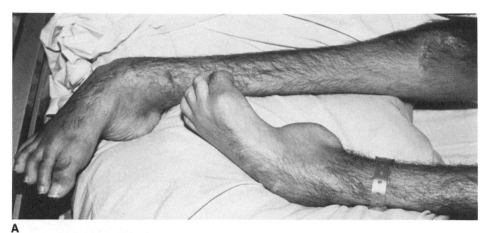

A

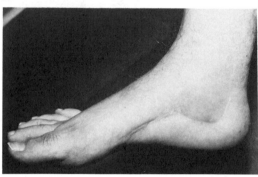

B

Fig. 8-8. **(A)** The foot of a patient who remained at a low level of neurologic recovery for 6 months. **(B)** The foot after plantar fasciectomy, posteriomedial release, and posterior tibialis tendon lengthening. Serial casts were necessary to correct the deformity.

This deformity may be primarily present or unmasked after the long toe flexors have been released (Fig. 8-9). A diagnostic posterior tibialis nerve block at the ankle joint helps differentiate between the long toe and short toe flexor muscles. This nerve block inhibits activity of the short toe flexors and should lessen or correct the deformity at the proximal interphalangeal joint but not true curling. The appropriate tendon release may be performed based on this block. No common tendon exists for the short toe flexors and each short flexor must be released individually at the toes.

Intrinsic Plus Deformity (Flexion of Metacarpophalangeal Joint and Extension of the Interphalangeal Joint)

Surgical indication: pain
Surgery: intrinsic release
Postoperative management: none

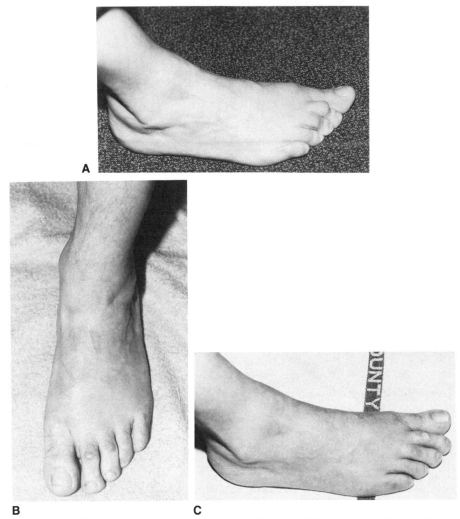

Fig. 8-9. **(A)** Short toe overactivity. Note the flexion of the proximal interphalangeal joint. **(B)** A procaine posterior tibialis nerve block at the ankle allows prediction of the proposed short toe flexor release. **(C)** The toes after short toe flexor releases have been performed.

This deformity is common in mild forms and is not often symptomatic. It may simulate a Babinski response. As the foot contacts the floor, the toes assume an intrinsic plus position (Fig. 8-10). The great toe may even go into extension but is usually asymptomatic. The intrinsic muscles are released through a dorsal incision at each metacarpophalangeal joint. Ambulation begins when pain and swelling subside.

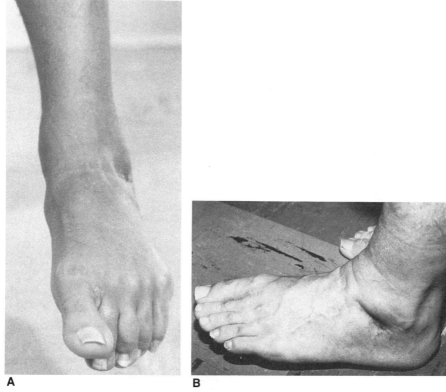

Fig. 8-10. **(A)** Intrinsic deformity of the common toes. **(B)** Toes after intrinsic release has been performed.

Toes, Foot, and Ankle

Equinovarus

Surgical indications: pain, orthotic containment, brace-free ambulation
Surgery: split anterior tibial tendon transfer (SPLATT), heel cord lengthening (TAL), and long toe flexor releases
Postoperative management: short leg walking cast for 6 weeks; ankle-foot orthosis (AFO) during he day and a posterior splint at night for 4 months

Equinovarus is the most common deformity of the lower extremity requiring surgical intervention (Fig. 8-11). Surgery combines three of the previously described procedures. Results are very predictable and very gratifying. Approximately 30 percent of our patients become brace-free after surgery.[8] This combined surgery allows many of the other patients to change AFOs from the heavy (shoe weight) metal double upright to a cosmetic, lightweight plastic AFO.

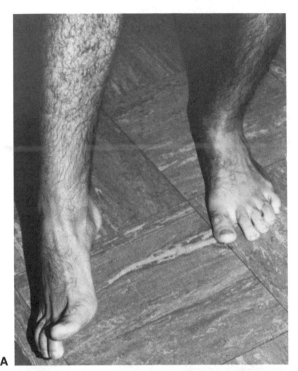

A

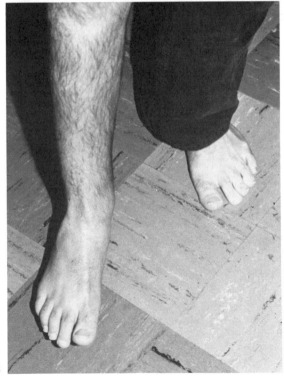

B

Fig. 8-11. (A) Classic equino-varus deformity of the lower extremity. (B) SPLATT, TAL, and long toe flexor releases have been performed. The patient was in a double metal upright AFO preoperatively. Postoperatively, a plastic AFO was necessary mainly because of ataxia.

Occasionally, this surgery allows conversion of a nonambulator to an ambulator. Finally, a small number of patients have improved wheelchair positioning and shoewear. Gait training begins in the short leg walking cast once pain and swelling have subsided. After 6 weeks, an AFO is used to control the foot during the day and a posterior splint at night. At 6 months after surgery, brace-free ambulation is attempted.

REFERENCES

1. Garland DE, Rhodes ME: Orthopedic management of brain-injured adults. Clin Orthop 131:111, 1978
2. Ough JL, Garland DE, Jordan C, Waters RL: Treatment of spastic joint contractures in mentally disabled adults. Orthop Clin North Am 12:143, 1981
3. Waters RL, Frazier J, Garland DE, Jordan C, Perry J: Electromyographic gait analysis before and after operative treatment for hemiplegic equinus and equinovarus deformity. J Bone Joint Surg 64A:284, 1982
4. Waters RL, Garland DE, Perry J, et al: Stiff-legged gait in hemiplegia: surgical correction. J Bone Joint Surg 61A:927, 1979
5. Waters RL, Perry J, Garland DE: Surgical correction of gait abnormalities following stroke. Clin Orthop 131:54, 1978
6. Waters RL, Garland DE: Acquired neurologic disorders of the adult foot. p. 325. In Mann RA (ed): Duvries Surgery of the Foot. 5th Ed. CV Mosby, St Louis, 1986
7. Waters RL, Garland DE: Disorders of the lower extremity in the stroke and head trauma patient. p. 2080. In Jahss MH (ed): Disorders of the Foot. 2nd Ed. WB Saunders, Philadelphia, 1991
8. Keenan MA, Creighton J, Garland DE, Moore T: Surgical correction of spastic equinovarus deformity in the adult head trauma patient. Foot Ankle 5:35, 1984
9. Perry J, Waters RL, Perrin T: Electromyographic analysis of equinovarus following stroke. Clin Orthop 131:47, 1978

9 | Reconstructive Surgery for Residual Upper Extremity Deformities

Douglas E. Garland

Surgery is performed less frequently in the upper extremity than in the lower extremity. Definitive surgical procedures should not be performed until $1\frac{1}{2}$ years after the initial head injury. Although a variety of deformities occur, improvement in function of the upper extremity is commonly not as dramatic as that achieved in the lower extremity. Observation of the upper extremity during use is an absolute necessity in the preoperative evaluation for functional surgery. Diagnostic procaine nerve blocks are very valuable in predicting surgical outcome and should be a part of the routine preoperative examination. The benefits of these blocks cannot be stressed enough. If available, dynamic electromyography further aids in the selection of proper tendon transfer, lengthening, or release.

NONFUNCTIONAL SURGERY

Surgery is most commonly indicated to lessen spasticity or correct deformities that are causing pain or preventing adequate hygiene. Nonfunctional procedures are occasionally necessary in the functional patient who has been neglected early after injury and has developed myostatic contractures. The following are the most common nonfunctional surgeries.

179

Shoulder

Adduction and Internal Rotation

Surgical indication: pain and hygiene
Surgery: release of the internal rotators of the shoulder
Postoperative management: vigorous passive range of motion

This was one of the more common deformities prior to widespread early rehabilitation and the emphasis on ranging of joints.[1] The deformity is presently uncommon (Fig. 9-1). There are four internal rotators of the shoulder: the pectoralis major, subscapularis, teres major, and latissimus dorsi muscles. If the deformity is mild, only the subscapularis and pectoralis major muscles are released. If the deformity is severe, all four muscles are released. The surgical approach is anteromedial and slightly inferior to the shoulder joint. Although full external rotation range is difficult to achieve and maintain, the pain subsides as well as the hygiene problems. Postoperatively, passive external rotation exercises are initiated when pain and swelling subside.

Subluxation

Surgical indication: pain, freedom from sling
Surgery: biceps sling (biceps tendon rerouted over clavicle)
Postoperative management: shoulder sling for 6 weeks

Subluxation of the shoulder is not common in this population (although it is common in strokes and some gunshot wounds to the head). Most shoulder subluxations are not painful; if there is pain, it frequently subsides within 6 months. A spastic biceps must be present for a good surgical result. The long biceps tendon is looped over the clavicle after resection of the distal end of the clavicle. This surgery consists of rerouting the biceps tendon without disturbing the origin and insertion of the biceps (Fig. 9-2). The transferred biceps tendon now has an increased mechanical advantage for reducing the shoulder subluxation. In effect, the rerouting relatively shortens the tendon, eliciting more tonus in the spastic biceps muscle. This relative increase in biceps spasticity causes shoulder reduction. In the past, tenodesis procedures about the shoulder have failed due to eventual attenuation of the transferred tendon. The patient is treated with a sling. No postoperative exercises are required.

Elbow

Flexion Contracture

Surgical indication: cosmesis, hygiene, and self-care
Surgery: musculocutaneous neurectomy; a concomitant elbow release if a fixed elbow contracture is greater than 75°
Postoperative management: serial or dropout casts for desired extension

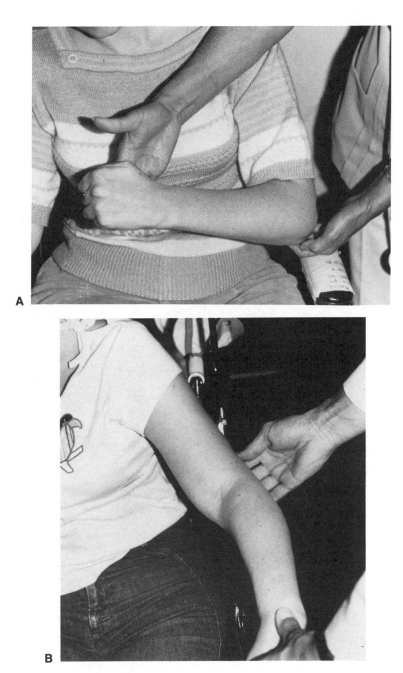

Fig. 9-1. (A) A patient with contracted internal rotators of the shoulder. Dressing and hygiene are rendered more difficult with this deformity. (B) The same patient after all four internal shoulder rotators have been released.

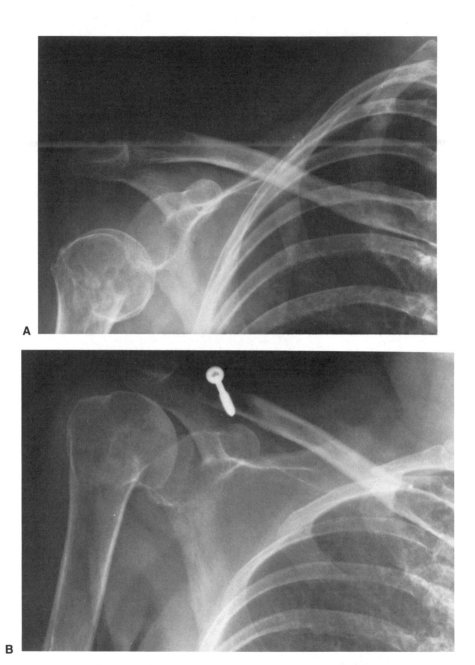

Fig. 9-2.   **(A)** Radiograph of a subluxated shoulder. The shoulder was painful. **(B)** Radiograph of the shoulder, which is now reduced after a bicipital sling procedure was performed.

Postoperative planning involves evaluation of brachioradialis muscle function.[2] Some brachioradialis activity, either active or spastic, must be present or an extension deformity will result postoperatively. An extension deformity may be as undesirable as a flexion deformity. A procaine musculocutaneous nerve block in the axilla or a brachial plexus block should be performed preoperatively. The nerve block decreases spasticity and allows evaluation of a fixed contracture. If the elbow lacks 75° or more of full extension, a concomitant elbow release is performed at surgery. If the nerve block is not performed preoperatively, elbow extension is evaluated after a muscle relaxant has been given at surgery to determine if an elbow release is indicated. A radiograph of the elbow must always be taken prior to the surgery to ensure that heterotopic ossification is not present. The musculocutaneous nerve is resected just distal to the shoulder (Fig. 9-3). An anterolateral approach to the elbow is utilized for the release of the flexors of the elbow and joint capsule if a flexion contracture of 75° or more was present. The anterolateral incision allows closure of the wound as the elbow is brought into extension and lessens the dead space, preventing hematoma formation and infection. A cylinder cast is applied at surgery with the elbow in maximum extension. Serial or dropout casts begin at 7 to 10 days and remain in use until the desired extension is achieved.

Wrist and Fingers

Flexion Contracture

Surgical indication: pain, hygiene, cosmesis
Surgery: sublimis to profundus transfer (STP) and ulnar motor neurectomy in the proximal hand
Postoperative management: platform type cast for three to six weeks

The STP is one of the most predictable procedures in the nonfunctional upper extremity.[3–5] Severe finger contractures are sometimes present, causing the fingernails to macerate the palm. Through the STP procedure, adequate lengthening of the finger flexors can be undertaken—without performing complete tenotomies of the flexor tendon—to achieve a neutral wrist and finger position. A muscle-tendon unit is left intact to prevent hyperextension. The sublimis tendons are transected near the carpal tunnel and the profundus tendons are severed near their muscle-tendon junction. The fingers and wrist are extended to a neutral position. Finger extension brings the profundus tendons into the wrist. They now lie near the sublimis motors and are sutured to them en masse. Suturing each tendon is difficult to perform, since it is impossible to set the proper tension for each finger individually. A Z-lengthening of the wrist and long thumb flexors is also undertaken. A deep motor ulnar neurectomy is also performed at the wrist to prevent intrinsic deformities, which are fre-

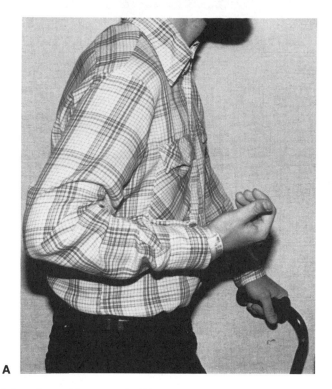

Fig. 9-3.   (A) A patient with cosmetically unacceptable spastic elbow flexion deformity. *(Figure continues.)*

quently unmasked by the STP procedure (Fig. 9-4). These hands occasionally require long-term platform splinting at night after the cast has been removed.

Wrist

Flexion Deformity (after STP)

Surgical indication: brace freedom or recurrence of wrist flexion contracture
Surgery: extensor wrist tenodesis or wrist fusion
Postoperative management: short arm cast for 6 to 12 weeks

This deformity may become evident after an STP procedure has been performed.[4] Persistent spastic wrist and finger flexors combined with poor finger extensor strength aid in the occurrence of the deformity. A tenodesis of the wrist using the wrist extensor muscles prevents the deformity. The extensor carpi radialis longus and brevis and the extensor carpi ulnaris tendons are split at their muscle-tendon junction. Drill holes are placed in the distal radius. The tendons are then passed through these drill holes and sutured on themselves.

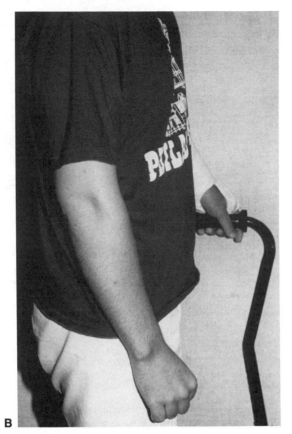

Fig. 9-3 *(Continued).* **(B)** A musculocutaneous neurectomy has been performed and the upper extremity has assumed a more natural posture. An elbow release was not necessary.

Fusion of the wrist is an acceptable alternative to wrist tenodesis. A short arm cast is applied until the tendons heal or the fusion unites.

Some patients with severe neurologic insult, especially the spastic quadriparetic patient, may have all these nonfunctional deformities in the same extremity.[6] These patients are excellent candidates for a combination of the above procedures in order to aid in their nursing care, to lessen the amount of ranging that the nursing home or family is performing, and to decrease the amount of splinting.

FUNCTIONAL SURGERY

Functional surgery is most predictable and beneficial when finger and wrist extensors are present at the hand and wrist but not functioning properly due to restriction by mild flexor wrist and finger spasticity or myostatic con-

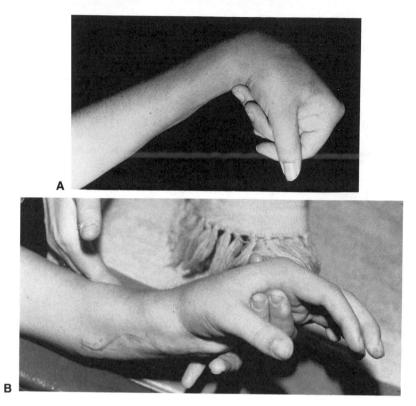

Fig. 9-4. **(A)** A hand with a severe flexion contracture. Hygiene is difficult. **(B)** A sublimus to profundus (STP) and ulnar motor neurectomy has been performed.

tracture.[6] Other important factors that help to produce good surgical results are average cognition and motivation, freedom from motor planning problems, spontaneous use, proximal limb control, no joint contractures, and two-point discrimination less than 10 mm. Stroke patients often have more control proximally with less control distally. The reverse frequently occurs in the head-injured. In the head-injured, hand control may demonstrate functional potential but placement may be impossible due to poor proximal control. Surgery to improve hand function is not indicated without first improving proximal control. Stroke patients frequently have significant impairment of sensation, militating against functional surgery, while the head-injury patient frequently has sensory sparing. Sometimes correctable deformities may exist and sensation may be present but motor planning problems prevent use even when the deformity is corrected. Preoperative observation during function is a "must," while diagnostic nerve blockers are a necessity.

Elbow

Clonic Elbow Flexors

Surgical indication: inability to extend arm smoothly
Surgery: selective release of the spastic flexor or flexors
Postoperative management: active range of motion

This dynamic deformity is uncommon. As the patient attempts to extend the elbow, cogwheel motion may be elicited. A dynamic electromyograph is necessary to identify the spastic or clonic elbow flexor. The offending muscle is surgically released near its insertion. Active range of motion is initiated when pain and swelling have subsided.

Wrist

Limited Extension

Surgical indication: improve hand function
Surgery: lengthen flexor carpi ulnaris and radialis muscles
Postoperative management: short arm cast for 3 weeks

This is one of the most common deformities in the functional upper extremity. Surgery frequently increases range of motion and function while improving cosmesis (Fig. 9-5). Procaine median and ulnar nerve blocks at the elbow allow evaluation of wrist extensor strength. Surgery is performed in the distal wrist. The flexor carpi radialis and ulnaris muscles are lengthened and the palmaris longus muscle is released. Active and passive ranging begins when the cast is removed at 3 weeks.

Limited Flexion

Surgical indication: improve hand function
Surgery: lengthen extensor carpi radialis longus and brevis muscles
Postoperative management: short arm cast for 3 weeks

This deformity is usually noted in patients with dystonic-type posturing. Hand function is less efficient in the dorsiflexed wrist (Fig. 9-6). Full finger extension is often difficult. Chronic wrist dorsiflexion encourages flexion contracture of the metacarpophalangeal joints. Degenerative joint disease of the carpal bones may occur when the deformity is left unchecked. Procaine radial nerve block allows prediction of surgical outcome. The wrist extensors may be lengthened at the tendons distally or by a muscle tendon slide (fractional

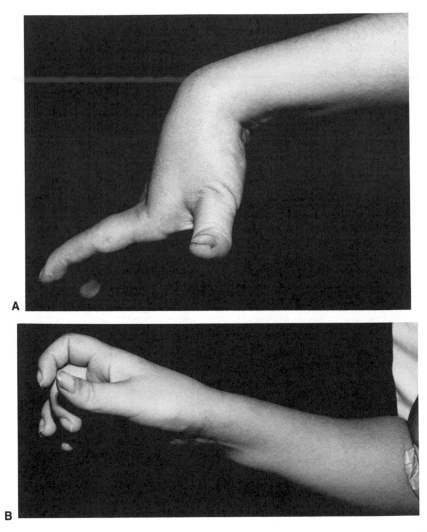

Fig. 9-5. **(A)** Voluntary hand opening. Finger extensors are obviously present. Functional potential of the wrist extensors is less obvious. **(B)** Median and ulnar procaine nerve blocks have been performed at the elbow. Wrist extensors are evident. *(Figure continues.)*

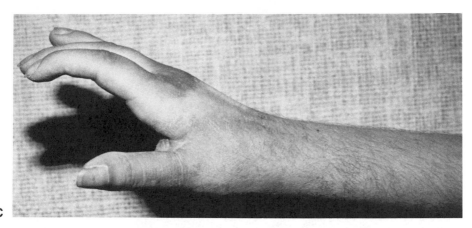

Fig. 9-5 *(Continued).* **(C)** The wrist flexors have been lengthened. A fractional lengthening of the finger flexors was also performed. Excellent hand positioning and function were obtained.

lengthening) more proximally. Active and passive ranging begins when the cast is removed.

Fingers

Limited Finger Extension

Surgical indication: improve hand opening
Surgery: fractional lengthening of flexor sublimis and profundus muscles
Postoperative management: short arm cast with bulky hand dressing for 3
    weeks

The deformity is frequently associated with spastic wrist flexors and surgery is frequently performed in conjunction with lengthening of the wrist flexors as well as of the flexor pollicis longus (Fig. 9-7). Procaine median and ulnar nerve blocks at the elbow allow prediction of surgical results and evaluation of extensor strength. The surgery is performed in the distal forearm. The proximal muscle tendon junctions are identified and transected.[4] The fingers are extended, causing the tendonous portion to slide distally on the remaining muscle fibers. Since a formal incision is not made into the tendons, suturing of the tendons to the muscles is not always necessary. Healing is rapid and some flexion motion is encouraged while the patient is in the cast. Fractional lengthening is technically easier and the outcome is more predictable than formal Z-lengthening of each finger flexor. If good finger and wrist extensor strength are evident, surgical results are often the most gratifying of the functional hand. Some active ranging begins in the bulky hand dressing.

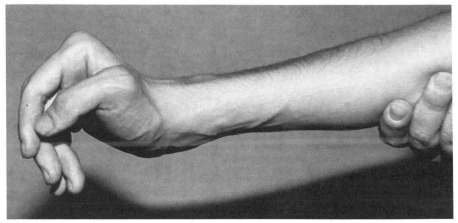

A

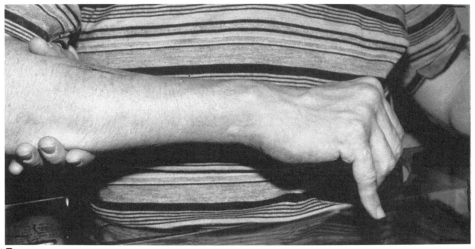

B

Fig. 9-6. **(A)** A hand with spastic wrist extensors. The chronically dorsiflexed position of the wrist encourages flexion contractures of the metacarpophalangeal joints. **(B)** The wrist extensors have been lengthened by a proximal muscle tendon slide (fractional lengthening). Hand position and use are greatly improved.

Limited Extension of the Distal Interphalangeal Joint

Surgical indication: increase hand opening

Surgery: fusion of the interphalangeal joint with release of the profundus tendons

Postoperative management: short arm cast for 3 weeks and Kirschner wires across the distal interphalangeal joint for 8 weeks

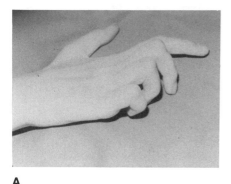
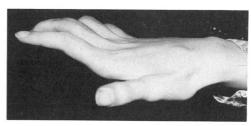

A   **B**

Fig. 9-7. (A) A fixed contracture is present at the proximal interphalangeal joints. (B) Considerable improvement in function is seen after a fractional lengthening of the sublimis and a collateral ligament resection at the proximal interphalangeal joints.

This deformity is not common. The profundus muscles are out of phase and are frequently active during both hand opening and closing. The sublimis muscles are in phase and are sufficient for hand closing. Chronic distal interphalangeal joint flexion interferes with grasp. The surgeon must decide to release the profundus tendon and fuse the distal interphalangeal joint or perform a fractional lengthening of the profundus tendons.

Flexion Contracture of the Proximal Interphalangeal Joint

Surgical indication: increase hand opening
Surgery: collateral ligament slide and fractional lengthening of the sublimis tendons (possibly profundus tendons)
Postoperative management: short arm cast plus Kirschner wires across the proximal interphalangeal joint for 3 weeks

This deformity is very uncommon. It develops from overactive sublimis flexors with limited ranging of the fingers after the head injury. The fingers assume a flexed position, especially at the proximal interphalangeal joint. The proximal interphalangeal joint is extended and the collateral ligament slides distally and adheres to the distal end of the proximal phalanx in a new position. The sublimis flexors and occasionally the profundus are weakened by fractional lengthening, preventing recurrence of the deformity and increasing hand opening. Active and passive ranging begins when the cast and Kirschner wires are removed.

Boutonniere

Surgical indication: increase grasp and hand opening
Surgery: lengthening of the sublimis muscles and of the lateral bands of the finger
Postoperative management: short arm cast and Kirschner wires across the distal and proximal interphalangeal joints for 6 weeks

This deformity is also uncommon. The boutonniere deformity consists of flexion of the proximal interphalangeal joints with hyperextension of the distal interphalangeal joints (Fig. 9-8). The deformity often results when active intrinsic muscles attempt to extend the fingers against spastic finger sublimis muscles. The lateral bands become attenuated, producing the deformity. Fractional lengthening of the sublimis muscles decreases the deforming force at the proximal interphalangeal joints. The lateral bands are usually contracted and must be lengthened to allow flexion at the distal interphalangeal joint Active and passive ranging begins when the cast and Kirschner wires are removed.

Intrinsic Plus

Surgical indication: increase hand opening
Surgery: intrinsic lengthening at the metacarpophalangeal joint
Postoperative management: Kirschner wires across the metacarpophalangeal joint for 3 to 6 weeks

Intrinsic plus deformities are common in the head-injured patient. A procaine ulnar nerve block at the wrist is helpful in making a diagnosis and allows prediction of the surgical results preoperatively, especially if phenol is to be employed. If this deformity is noted during acute rehabilitation, phenol ulnar motor nerve injection in the palm often prevents late deformities. This allows continued therapy and prevents intrinsic plus contractures. If the phenol nerve block is successful and a recurrence of deformity occurs, consideration of a complete motor neurectomy of the ulnar motor branch in the palm may be entertained. If the deformity is fixed, individual Z-lengthening of the collateral ligaments at the metacarpophalangeal joint is performed. Hand opening is improved but full metacarpophalangeal extension is uncommon. Active and passive ranging begins when the Kirschner wires are removed.

Thumb

Three basic thumb deformities occur. The "thumb in palm" may be secondary to a spastic flexor pollicis longus muscle (Fig. 9-9A). Second, the deformity may be due to spasticity of the adductor muscles of the thumb (Fig. 9-9B). Last, it may result from spastic thenar muscles of the thumb (Fig. 9-9C).

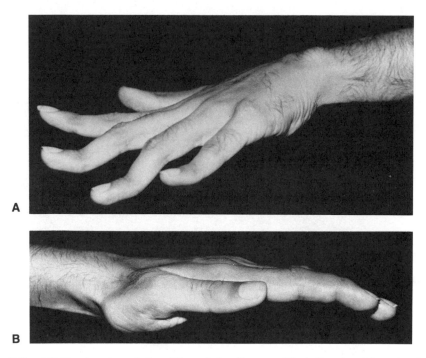

Fig. 9-8. (A) Boutonniere deformities of the fingers. (B) A fractional lengthening of the sublimis and lengthening of the lateral bands has improved use.

The deformities may be dynamic or fixed (Fig. 9-9D). They may also occur from a singular deforming force or in combinations. These deformities can be differentiated by physical examination and differential procaine nerve blocks. Hyperflexion of the interphalangeal joint is secondary to the long thumb flexor. Median and ulnar nerve blocks at the wrist will not correct this deformity, since the long thumb flexor is innervated more proximally. A median nerve block at the elbow allows correction of the deformity. If the deformity is the result of thenar muscle spasticity, a procaine block of the median nerve at the wrist permits correction of the deformity. If the deformity is secondary to the adduction deformity, the deformity will be lessened by a procaine ulnar nerve block at the wrist. Fixed deformities will not be corrected by any nerve block.

Thumb in Palm

Surgical indication: increase thumb opening
Surgery: release of the adductor at its origin or its insertion
Postoperative management: thumb spica cast for 3 weeks

The diagnosis of a spastic adductor muscle is confirmed by ulnar nerve block at the wrist. The adductor muscle may be recessed at its insertion on the

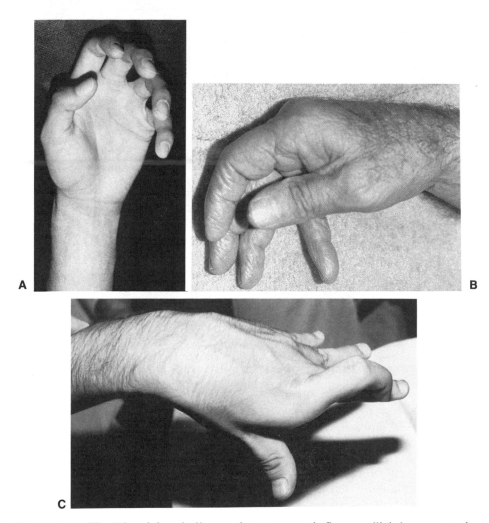

Fig. 9-9.   (A) The "thumb in palm" secondary to a spastic flexor pollicis longus muscle. (B) The "thumb in palm" secondary to the adductors of the thumb. (C) The "thumb in palm" secondary to the spastic thenars of the palm. *(Figure continues.)*

thumb or a muscle slide of the adductor muscle from its origin in the palm may be performed. A first web space contracture is often associated with the deformity. If the deformity is associated with a web space contracture, a Z-lengthening of the skin in the web space and a release of the adductor pollicis muscle at its insertion in the thumb is performed (Fig. 9-10). Active and passive ranging begins when the cast is removed.

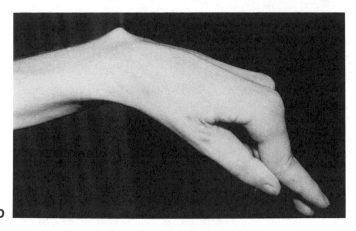

Fig. 9-9 *(Continued).* **(D)** Fixed "thumb in palm" with soft tissue contracture.

Thumb in Palm

Surgical indication: increase thumb opening
Surgery: release of the thenar muscles at their insertion or muscle slide from their origin
Postoperative management: thumb spica cast for 3 weeks

The diagnosis is confirmed by a median nerve block at the wrist. If deformity is mild, the short thumb flexor muscle is recessed at its insertion. If the

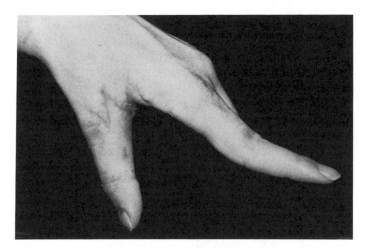

Fig. 9-10.   A Z-lengthening of the skin in the first web space along with a release of the adductor muscle at its insertion has allowed improved opening of the thumb in Figure 9-9D.

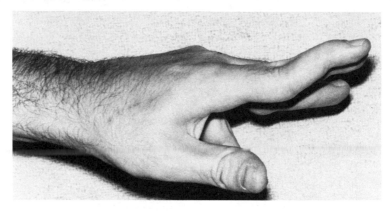

Fig. 9-11. A release of the origin of the thenar muscles in the palm has been performed on the hand in Figure 9-9C.

deformity is severe or if it is associated with an adduction contracture, a release of the origin of these muscles is performed in the palm, allowing them to slide distally (Fig. 9-11). Active and passive ranging begins when the cast is removed.

Thumb in Palm

Surgical indication: increased hand opening
Surgery: lengthening of flexor pollicis longus and fusion of interphalangeal joint
Postoperative management: thumb spica cast for 6 weeks

The diagnosis is confirmed by a median nerve block at the wrist. The deformity results from a spastic long thumb flexor. The long thumb extensor is not strong enough to extend the distal joint. Fusion of the interphalangeal joint at the time of the thumb flexor lengthening allows more advantageous use of the short thumb extensor. Active and passive ranging begins when the cast and Kirschner wire are removed.

REFERENCES

1. Braun RM, West F, Mooney V, et al: Surgical treatment of the painful shoulder contracture in the stroke patient. J Bone Joint Surg 53A:1307, 1971
2. Garland DE, Thompson R, Waters RL: Musculocutaneous neurectomy for spastic elbow flexion in nonfunctional upper extremities in adults. J Bone Joint Surg 1:108, 1980
3. Braun RM, Vise GT, Roper B: Preliminary experience with superficialis to profundus tendon transfer in the hemiplegic upper extremity. J Bone Joint Surg 56A:466, 1974

4. Waters RL: Upper extremity surgery in stroke patients. Clin Orthop 131:30, 1978
5. Ough JL, Garland DE, Jordan C, Waters RL: Treatment of spastic joint contracture in mentally disabled. Orthop Clin North Am 12:143, 1981
6. Waters RL, Garland DE, Nickel VL: Upper extremity surgery in stroke patients. p. 466. In Lamb DW, Kuczynski K (eds): 2nd Ed. Practice of Hand Surgery. Blackwell Scientific Publications, Edinburgh, Scotland, 1989

10 | Strategies for Community Integration

Mitchell Rosenthal
John F. O'Leary

Traumatic brain injury, regardless of severity, often poses significant challenges to the injured person for successfully becoming integrated into the home, family, and community. Despite the heroic and remarkably effective efforts of most acute care neurotrauma and neurorehabilitation teams, the individual who has suffered a brain injury is not typically able to leave the hospital within days or weeks to resume a normal lifestyle. Injury to the brain resulting in prolonged periods of unconsciousness, and neurologic disruption leads to a wide variety of neurobehavioral deficits.[1] The nature and extent of these deficits, in combination with the physical sequelae, can place great limitations on the coping abilities of both the brain-injured survivor and the family members. Thus, discharge from the inpatient rehabilitation unit is often followed by continued treatment in a variety of settings to optimize the capacity of the newly brain-injured person to become a productive member of the community.

In recent years, the World Health Organization[2] has provied a basis for understanding the nature of disability following catastrophic illness or injury. In this scheme, sometimes referred to as the Impairment, Disability, Handicap (IDH) model, a disease or disorder may lead to a loss of organ structure or function—that is, an *impairment*. This may then lead to a diminution of the person's capacity to effectively perform certain aspects of daily living—that is, a *disability*. In turn, this will lead to a disadvantage for the person in fulfilling normal social roles—a *handicap*. More specifically, the WHO defines *handicap*

199

as including six key aspects of role function: orientation, physical independence, mobility, occupation, social integration, and economic self-sufficiency. The focus of this chapter will be on the handicap resulting from traumatic brain injury and various ways of understanding, measuring, and reducing it.

CONTINUUM OF CARE

The need for continued therapeutic services following acute rehabilitation for traumatic brain injury has resulted in a proliferation of treatment options in the community.[3] In addition to the traditional outpatient therapy performed in the rehabilitation hospital or clinic, specialized treatment options have been developed for persons with brain injury who are seeking to optimize community reentry skills (Table 10-1). In fact, this explosion in post–acute programming has led the Commission on Accreditation of Rehabilitation Facilities[4] to adopt a set of brain injury standards applying exclusively to "community-integrated programs." These standards provide guidelines for community reentry programs; they include administration, marketing, ethics, staffing, programming, program evaluation, education, and training of personnel. To assist persons with brain injuries and their families in making decisions about posthospital care, the case manager role has become an increasingly important professional in the discharge planning process. Case managers may be internal (e.g., social workers within the referring or receiving program) or external (e.g., within an insurance company or a social service or vocational rehabilitation agency). Regardless of the source of case management services, this individual needs to have the knowledge and skills to fairly and effectively guide persons with brain injuries and their families to the best community reentry option among a variety of possibilities.

Of the options listed in Table 10-1, there may be a significant overlap in therapeutic approach in these programs. Perhaps the most common model is the day treatment approach. In this model, persons with brain injury attend a treatment program (usually within the community rather than in the hospital) that provides coordinated intensive therapy for approximately 4 to 6 hours per day. This treatment is delivered by an interdisciplinary team of rehabilitation professionals (e.g., physician, physical, occupational and speech therapists, psychologist/neuropsychologist, driver-education specialist, recreational thera-

Table 10-1. Types of Community Reentry Programs

Outpatient therapy
Home health care
Day hospital or day treatment
Transitional living
Residential neurobehavioral treatment
Special education
Vocational training
Supported living
Independent living

pist, and vocational counselor), with a stronger emphasis on the psychosocial than on the medical approach. Involvement of family or significant others is critical and is incorporated into the treatment plan. Treatment often lasts at least 3 to 6 months and tends to be functionally oriented, with a significant amount of treatment occurring in actual community settings (i.e., supermarket, bank, shopping center). This model will be the basis of the examples provided in the rest of the chapter, though many of the same principles apply to other treatment models.

COMPONENTS OF COMMUNITY INTEGRATION

The process of community reentry can take several different forms, depending on the pattern and speed of recovery, availability of community treatment options, access to transportation, and financial sponsorship. For example, the individual could enter a community-based treatment program as a component of the post–acute discharge plan. This approach would essentially constitute what has traditionally been referred to as outpatient treatment. In another example, if residential placement (i.e., transitional living) is needed because of either physical or cognitive limitations, community reentry could begin in a more structured fashion, including the provision of extensive supervision. In other cases, the brain injury survivor may not have received sufficient treatment at the outset or have failed to effectively maintain independent living function over time. It is not unusual to see "older" cases recycling through the system because of current problems associated with changes in their level of independent functioning.

Regardless of the nature of the referral or the historical stage of the injury, there appear to be consistent components for all potential candidates for community reintegration programming. These include the following candidate selection and treatment considerations.

Establishing Functional Treatment Goals

If a community reentry program is to be effective, it must have clearly understandable goals that can serve as targets for the treatment, as a motivational impetus for the patient, and as a means of comparing treatment outcome with initial expectations. These goals are usually identified in terms of accomplishments or outcomes that a patient wants or needs in order to function more independently at home, at school, on a job, or within the social network of the immediate neighborhood. The nature of the functional goals provides the essential bridge between the clinical interventions of rehabilitation and the practice carryover of those gains in the daily activity pattern of the individual. For example, ambulation exercises within the clinic take on a new perspective when practiced in varying community settings—such as community parks, shopping centers, restaurants, and sports stadiums—where distance, terrain, accessibility, and distractions can be confounding variables. In addition, by extending the clinic into the community, therapy can take on much more intrinsic value for the patient, generating motivation to persist at difficult treatment tasks and to improve in a consistent fashion. The use of functional, measurable treatment goals also provides the rehabilitation team with useful information about the efficacy of the treatment being provided. Outcome data can easily be obtained simply by comparing initial baseline measurements with subsequent gains in functional activities. In this way justification for treatment, assessment of outcome effectiveness and predictions about future needs for treatment can be more definitive.

Capacity for Learning

"Learning potential" can be an elusive ingredient in the rehabilitation process. However, it is a crucial element for the clinician to understand in defining a treatment program. This is because *all* rehabilitation interventions, irrespective of discipline, can best be considered as retraining or relearning interventions. This is clearly evident in working with persons with traumatic brain injury where impaired memory is often an identifiable cognitive component. However, "memory impairment" alone is insufficient to define what an individual's learning potential is or could be. One patient could be amnestic and still learn, while another might have an unimpaired memory and not learn. Rather, learning potential includes a combination of factors such as the preserved components of the individual's memory, the intrinsic value of the treatment goal (i.e., walking), or the social support for following through on a treatment goal.

The first of these components, the identification of the preserved components of an individual's memory, is often clarified in the neuropsychological evaluation and through empirical learning trials done within the clinical setting. The neuropsychological examination can elucidate the integrity of basic memory and learning functions, including the ability for sustained concentration, the consolidation process of short-term memory, the ease of recall from long-term storage, and the need for various forms of cuing to facilitate the recall of previously learned information. The neuropsychological examination should also be able to identify the individual's potential for incidental learning, which occurs at a more implicit level. This is sometimes referred to as "automatic" learning because it often involves remembering information or sequences which one did not consciously attempt to remember. In some clinical cases, the use of implicit or automatic learning may be the primary mode of intervention, based on the extent of impairment in other aspects of the person's memory. As a result, information about a person's cognitive ability and memory functions can help the clinician to use instruction incorporating the cognitive strengths of the person receiving treatment.

In addition to the status of the patient's learning potential, it is also useful to try a series of small empirical experiments designed to test any clinical "hunches" the therapist may have about what the patient is capable of doing or learning. Examples of this may include chaining a sequence of exercises together to elicit a more automatic form of learning or asking for a verbal description or a nonverbal demonstration of exercise patterns previously reviewed in earlier sessions. In this way, the therapist can "test" certain hypotheses about how the patient may best retain what is being taught from one session to the next. This is particularly important in those cases where there appears to be inconsistent carryover from one session to the next or where the nature of the cognitive limitations is becoming a major hurdle to any treatment gains.

The second major factor in defining a patient's learning potential involves the intrinsic *value* of the therapy goals. This can be a very potent but difficult-to-define influence on the course of treatment. Nevertheless, the importance of clarifying ways to optimize client motivation as an aspect of treatment cannot be overemphasized. In addition, the use of highly valued goals (such as walking) can often be used to improve the perceived merit of less valued goals (such as repetitive drills for strengthening or endurance building) by linking one to the other. That is, the therapist links highly valued tasks to less valued ones, making attention to the former contingent upon completion of the latter—which, although less valued, may be therapeutically necessary exercises. Such an approach can enhance the whole treatment program.

The third major component in defining learning potential involves the extent of social support for carryover beyond the therapy session. The more consistently the caregivers follow through on the identified treatment program, the more likely it is that treatment gains will generalize and be maintained. It should be noted, however, that given the concreteness of many persons with brain injury, generalization of treatment effects may be quite elusive. The involvement of the family members or caregivers in the treatment process will be best facilitated if it occurs early and is identified as a "reasonable and necessary" component of treatment. In this way, the involvement of the patient's social support system is defined as an expected, rather than an ancillary, aspect of treatment.

Termination of Treatment

The process of effective treatment in the postacute setting can clearly be facilitated if an end point to treatment is established at the start of therapy. This allows for the definition of a target or direction for the treatment. Clinical management problems that arise during the postacute phase often involve some problem with how or when treatment should end. As a result, termination issues are better managed at the beginning rather than closer to the time of discharge.

The clinical case lore on this issue is unlimited. For example, it is not unusual to find oneself working with patients who want either to leave treatment too early or to stay too long. Either situation can be frustrating for the therapist attempting to return the patient to the most effective level of functioning. With "older" cases, treatment issues often revolve around outcome expectations that may or may not be realistic. As a result, it is very important to define the parameters of treatment from the start, including the time lines for the length of treatment, in order to avoid conflict over the expected length or outcome of treatment.

Conceptual Issues

Community integration may often involve some form of formal cognitive rehabilitation.[5] There are many ways in which this form of rehabilitation intervention is defined and implemented. Some clinicians and researchers have suggested that none of the currently used terms (i.e., cognitive rehabilitation, neurorehabilitation, community integration) conjure up a specific set of techniques or treatment approaches. Nevertheless, it is important to be familiar with some broad, working definitions of the terms *cognitive rehabilitation* and *community integration* so as to understand how the conceptual framework of each term drives the intervention process.

Cognitive rehabilitation generally involves improving the patient's cognitive capacity for effectively responding to multisensory input (from hearing, vision, touch, and proprioception) in an efficient manner and for improving problem-solving abilities in effective daily functioning. *Community integration* incorporates various forms of *cognitive rehabilitation* but places the focus of treatment on the use of community settings for "real-life" training. It is essentially an umbrella concept, subsuming various rehabilitation interventions as components of this approach.

In more specific terms, Fryer and Fralish[6] identified three broad treatment approaches within this field of rehabilitation, each implying a different set of basic assumptions about the nature of the work. The first of these is the *instrumental skills approach*, which does not make any assumptions about improving the cognitive deficits identified through evaluation. Rather, treatment is approached from a skills development standpoint with no direct focus on actual cognitive remediation as a treatment goal. The second treatment approach is just the reverse. *The hierarchical task approach* has cognitive remediation as its central focus, and treatment is organized around a theoretical hierarchy of increasingly complex cognitive tasks. The third treatment approach is referred to as the *functional activities approach*. It essentially uses daily activities as the mode of intervention, with training centered on mastering those tasks which will allow a person to return to live and work in the least restrictive setting.

There are limitations to each of these approaches considered alone; most cognitive rehabilitation specialists employ some combination of all three. However, it is important to keep in mind that this is a field of rehabilitation which lacks a sound theoretical base. As a result, clinicians need to monitor their clinical practices empirically by using a hypothesis-testing approach in their daily work to assess basic diagnostic assumptions as well as carryover outside of therapy and into the home or community setting. In this way, efficacy is based on results—and not merely on the presumptions or theoretical orientation of the clinician or treatment program.

Diagnostic Considerations

Persons with brain injury referred to a community integration program may or may not have their diagnostic status clarified at the time of admission. It is usually customary to conduct some form of initial assessment in order to ascertain which key motor and cognitive skills exist at the time of admission and which are impaired. This is also the time to select intervention techniques and the appropriate sequence of treatment objectives by means of exploratory diagnostic therapy. The actual therapeutic approaches involving neurodevelopmental intervention,[7] proprioceptive neuromuscular facilitation,[8] neurorehabilitation,[9,10] and sensory integration[11] are all well documented in the physical therapy literature. However, additional diagnostic considerations must include other areas as well (Table 10-2).

In reviewing these considerations, *community mobility* could involve the use of adaptive aids and techniques. However, technologically complex such adaptive devices may be, the "patient/device fit" is a crucial component for ensuring effective use of such assistive devices. This begins with the introduction of the equipment to the patient and family, which should be paced in order to optimize the chances of successful use. The motoric, communicative, cognitive, emotional, and situational requirements of using a device should be analyzed carefully during this phase, with the demands graded to the patient's level of ability. This type of approach is more likely to promote early incorporation of any assistive devices and to decrease the probability that such equipment will become a "closet" item because the patient or family feel too annoyed or challenged by the device. In any event, mobility interventions that generate early experiences of *success* are much more likely to carry over into the home and community.

Considerations regarding community placement often revolve around some assessment of the patient's endurance, cognitive and physical flexibility, and physical strength. In addition to formal clinical assessments of these levels, daily activities—either at home or within the community—can often provide significant information about actual levels, because the factors of familiarity and interest are not generally sources of interference. That is, the familiarity of home or a community setting can often elicit more automatic responses (which can control for the novelty of some clinical assessment procedures)

Table 10-2. Important Diagnostic Considerations

1. Capability for community mobility
2. Potential for sustained activity requiring endurance, strength, or flexibility
3. Ability to maintain behavioral control over any behaviors identified as excessive, socially inappropriate, or physically inefficient
4. Potential for independent living in a safe and effective manner (including any needs for supervision)
5. Capability for competitive employment and/or potential to return to school
6. Ability to reestablish satisfying social and leisure activities
7. Awareness of deficits

while also generating interest in doing more activity because of the "normalizing" effect of a community setting.

These "normal" settings also provide ample opportunities for assessing the ability to control behaviors that have been deemed to be excessive, socially inappropriate, or physically inefficient. Given the high value attached to "normal" (as in familiar, nonclinical) activities by most patients, the nature of any significant control problems will be much more apparent when they are displayed within such a desired setting. This is the real diagnostic and treatment value of using community settings for behavioral management concerns.

Therapists are often called upon to state a position on issues related to supervision, safety, and potential for independent living. Rather than relying on supposition or conjecture, therapists must test this issue within the environment in which the patient will live following discharge. This provides the best setting in which to assess the potential for independent living or any ongoing supervision needs.

Similarly, the assessment of vocational and educational potential can best be made within the context of work or school trials, which illustrate by demonstration what a patient's actual capabilities may be within a given work or school context. While this may appear obvious to many clinicians, it is also not unusual within this field for some therapists to answer such questions based on the results of physical and cognitive test results alone. However, the ecological validity of many of our current formal test procedures remains limited, and this underscores the need for in situ trials, or practice opportunities. The same guidelines are pertinent for reestablishing satisfying social and leisure activities.

Finally, the "awareness-of-deficits factor" has received increasing attention within the past few years.[12,13] This inability to acknowledge the presence or severity of deficits caused by impaired brain function can be a major obstacle to post–acute care or community integration treatment. If this is identified as a problem in the diagnostic process, strategies must be clearly identified to increase awareness of deficits and thus to improve the likelihood of a successful outcome for the treatment program. In some cases, severe unawareness or denial of deficits may be a reason for declining to accept an individual into a community integration program.

Course of Treatment

Treatment, within this context, begins with the identification of the goals (or purpose) of treatment. This allows for clarification of where the treatment program will head and enjoins the patient to sign on to the program both literally and figuratively. In addition to identifying outcome goals, an estimated length of treatment is provided at this time to lend some perspective to the amount of time that it will take to reach the identified goals. By establishing both an expected outcome and a time limit, the community integration program is given definition and focus. The practice of having the patient, family, and team sign the initial treatment plan and monthly progress reports allows for both greater agreement on the nature of the treatment plan and mutual understanding about the roles, expectations, and focus of the clinical program. It also fits into recent revisions in accreditation guidelines, which require written documentation and acceptance of the treatment plan. Many case management problems can be circumvented or contained by establishing greater mutual understanding between the patient and/or family and the treatment team at the start of the program.

In addition to these initial strategies, the treatment course generally involves some combination of new learning that must be data-based and geared toward generalization outside of treatment. Szekeres and colleagues[14] identified seven general principles of intervention having broad application within a community integration program. These are:

1. The generation of success is crucial to facilitating patient progress and rebuilding a productive self-concept. This is more likely to occur when the treatment task difficulty, performance expectations, and application of compensation techniques are controlled in a way that builds a sense of accomplishment and self-esteem.

2. All treatment tasks involve systematically graduated demands designed to increase broad cognitive and physical capabilities in the areas of efficiency, level, and scope and manner of performance, with the focus on transferring those improvements to the conditions of daily life.

3. Meaningful learning occurs through habituation and generalization training. Instruction in the transfer of skills from one setting to another may be necessary.

4. In order to generate functional independence and increased motivation, the treating clinicians must encourage patients to participate in the goal-setting process, help in planning meaningful treatment activities, and assist in solving problems. Passive participants reduce their chances for successful community reentry.

5. Consistency of expectations among both the treating clinicians and patient's family facilitates the potential for effective new learning and the generalization of treatment.

6. Personal characteristics—such as age, pretrauma social, educational, and vocational status, as well as current levels of cognitive functioning—must be considered in designing treatment tasks.

7. Group therapy can provide a highly useful intervention approach, especially within the context of community integration programming, in which social judgment and interactive skills are employed in ways that allow for modeling, constructive feedback, and peer encouragement.

Ultimately, the best measures of the success of therapy lie with demonstrated improvement in family and other social relationships and a return to some level of productivity.

Evaluation of Outcome

In this era of cost containment in health care, the burden of demonstrating the cost-effectiveness of post–acute brain injury rehabilitation is clearly present. As Johnston and Lewis[15] have noted, the relationship between costs of post–acute brain injury rehabilitation and achievement of successful outcomes is far from clear.

Unlike acute rehabilitation, there is no "universally accepted" gauge of success—such as the Functional Independence Measure, which is used widely to assess program effectiveness. Each community integration program, particularly those in compliance with CARF accreditation guidelines, has its own system guidelines and program evaluation instruments, but often without any proven reliability or validity. Methodologic issues—such as validity of patient self-report versus observer ratings, relationship between preinjury status and postinjury behavior, and weighting of items—must also be confronted.

Several noteworthy approaches have recently been published. Malec and colleagues[16] reported the use of goal-attainment methodology in a post–acute brain injury rehabilitation program. This method calls for highly individualized goals to be established and progress to be measured against *them*—as opposed to the evaluation of performance against an arbitrary standard or societal norm. The study examined the use of the instrument with a sample of 82 brain-injured patients enrolled in a post–acute community integration program. Significant improvements were found in supervision and care requirements, employment, and daily activity after participation in the program. Another instrument, known as the Community Integration Questionnaire (CIQ), was recently developed by Willer and colleagues.[17] This 15-item instrument, designed to be administered to either the survivor of brain injury or family member in person or over the telephone, has shown initial good test-retest reliability (0.91 to 0.97) and internal consistency (0.76). A factor analysis yielded three factors or subscales identified as home integration, social integration, and productive activity. In initial studies, it was found to significantly differentiate between nondisabled controls and brain-injured patients at 1 year postinjury.

CONCLUSION

Community reentry programming for persons with brain injury has been in existence for only a decade but has become a key element in the continuum of care. The expansion of treatment options and programs has thus far exceeded the empirical data that would confirm the efficacy or cost-effectiveness of these approaches.

In this chapter, a model of community reentry emphasizing functional, measurable client-centered treatment has been advanced. Factors such as preinjury history, physical and cognitive impairment, family dynamics, financial and environmental limitations, and awareness of deficits are important considerations for the physical therapist working in the context of a community reentry treatment program. Careful diagnostic assessment and an individualized treatment plan that recognizes the person's values, motivations, and needs are important ingredients for success. Finally, it seems clear that more scientifically rigorous methods of program evaluation and measurement of outcome will have to be developed, widely used, and disseminated if community reentry programs are to continue to flourish.

ACKNOWLEDGEMENTS

Preparation of this manuscript was supported, in part, by grant H133A20016 from the National Institute on Disability and Rehabilitation Research, United States Department of Education.

REFERENCES

1. Rosenthal M, Griffith ER, Bond MR, Miller JD (eds): Rehabilitation of the Adult and Child with Traumatic Brain Injury. FA Davis, Philadelphia, 1989
2. World Health Organization: Classification of Impairments, Disabilities and Handicaps. World Health Organization, Geneva, Switzerland, 1980
3. Cervelli L: Reentry into the community and systems of post-hospital care. p. 463. In Rosenthal M, Griffith ER, Bond MR, Miller JD (eds): Rehabilitation of the Adult and Child with Traumatic Brain Injury, 2nd Ed. FA Davis, Philadelphia, 1990
4. Commission on Accreditation of Rehabilitation Facilities: Brain Injury Standards: Community Integrated Programs. Commission on Accreditation of Rehabilitation Facilities, Tucson, AZ, 1988, 1993
5. Kreutzer JS, Wehman P: Community Integration Following Traumatic Brain Injury. Paul Brookes, Baltimore, MD, 1990
6. Fryer J, Fralish K: Cognitive rehabilitation. p. 7-1. In Deutsch PM, Fralish KB (eds): Innovations in Head Injury Rehabilitation. Matthew Bender, Albany, NY, 1989
7. Bobath B: Adult Hemiplegia: Evaluation and Treatment. 2nd Ed. Heinemann, London, 1978
8. Knott M, Voss DE: Proprioceptive Neuromuscular Facilitation. Harper & Row, New York, 1968
9. Farber SD: Neurorehabilitation: A Multi-Sensory Approach. WB Saunders, Philadelphia, 1982
10. Umphred DA: Neurological Rehabilitation. CV Mosby, St Louis, 1985
11. Ayres AJ: The Development of Sensory Integration Theory and Practice. Kendall/Hunt Publishing, Dubuque, IA, 1974
12. Crosson B, Barco PP, Bolesta MM et al: Awareness and compensation in postacute head injury rehabilitation. J Head Trauma Rehab 4:46, 1989
13. Prigatano GP, Altman IM: Impaired awareness of behavioral limitations after traumatic brain injury. Arch Phy Med Rehab 71:1058, 1990
14. Szekeres SF, Ylvisaker M, Cohen SB: A framework for cognitive rehabilitation therapy. p. 122. In Ylvisaker M, Gobble EM (eds): Community Re-Entry for Head Injured Adults. College Hill, San Diego, CA, 1987

15. Johnston MV, Lewis F: Outcomes of community re-entry programs for brain injury survivors. Brain Inj 5:141, 1991
16. Malec JF, Smigelski JS, DePompolo R: Goal attainment scaling and outcome measurement in post acute brain injury rehabilitation. Arch Phy Med Rehab 72:138, 1991
17. Willer B, Rosenthal M, Kreutzer JS et al: Assessment of community integration following rehabilitation for traumatic brain injury. J Head Trauma Rehab 8:75, 1993

Index

Page number followed by f *indicate figures; those followed by* t *indicate tables.*

Activities of Daily Living (ADL), brain injury
    effects on, 34, 34t
Acute care, following head injury, 1–31. *See also*
    Head injury(ies), acute care hospital
    management of.
Adduction contracture, of the hip, nonfunctional
    surgery for, 162–163
Adduction of the shoulder, nonfunctional surgery
    for, 180, 181f
Airway(s), management of, in head-injured patients,
    3, 5
Ankle
    bones of, 139, 140f
    mobilization of, 142–146, 144f–147f. *See also*
        Mobilization, ankle and foot.
    problems of, case studies, 147–160, 149f–159f
    residual deformities of, surgery for, 166, 168,
        175–176, 177f
Ankle-foot orthosis (AFO), 88–89
    case studies, 147–160, 149f–159f
    designing of
        assessment of ankle and foot for, 139
        guidelines for, 141–142
    dorsal, 151, 155f, 156f
    fabrication of, assessment of ankle and foot for,
        139
    modifications over time, 142
    postural grounding with, 138–139
    purpose of, 137
Ankle positioning, in wheelchair seating, 134–135
Aphasia, handicaps related to, 34t
Arterial lines, in head-injured patients, 7
Ativan, indications for and actions of, 5t

Baclofen, indications for and actions of, 5t
Bedside table, uses of, 25, 27f
Behavior
    motor. *See* Motor behavior.
    skilled, definition of, 43

Behavioral impairment, following brain injury,
    35–37, 36t
Behavioral treatment strategies, 39–42, 40t, 41f
Block(s)
    chemical substances used in, 89
    definition of, 89
    indications for, 89
Bobath ball, uses of, 25, 25f
Bones, of ankle and foot, 139, 140f
Botulinim toxin, for spasticity, 92
Boutonniere deformities, nonfunctional surgery for,
    192, 193f
Brain injury(ies)
    acute rehabilitation following, community
        integration following, 199–209. *See also*
        Community integration.
    cognitive categories following, 37–38
    heterotopic ossification following, 92–96
    impairments following, 34, 34t
        behavioral, 35–37, 36t
        cognitive, 35–37, 36t
        swallowing, 99–115. *See also* Swallowing
        dysfunction.
    joint contractures following, 79
    learning ability affected by, 43
    physical categories following, 38
    rehabilitation following. *See also* Head injury(ies)
        and specific types of rehabilitation, e.g.,
        Cognitive rehabilitation; Motor control,
        restoration of.
    process of, 33
    spasticity following, 80–81, 89–92
        botulinim toxin for, 92
    spontaneous recovery from, 56
    surgery following, 91–92
    wheelchair seating and positioning for patients
        with, 117–136. *See also* Wheelchair seating.
    WHO classification of, 34, 34t
Bupivacaine, for spasticity, 89–91
Butler, R., 2

Care, acute, following head injury, 1–31. *See also* Head injury(ies), acute care hospital management of.

Cast(s)
dropout, 83–85, 84f
fiberglass, 83
indications for, 83t
inhibitive, 85
misapplication of, skin breakdown due to, 86
outrigger devices for, 85
plaster of Paris, 83
resting, 82
serial, versus dynamic splints, 86–87
spreader bars for, 85
strip, with bilateral toe-spreaders, 156
types of, 83t

Cast brace, 85

Casting
for ankle-foot orthosis, 156, 157f–159f
in head-injured patients, 21–22
inhibitive, 85
serial
benefits of, 82
cast application, 82–86, 84f
considerations in, 82
indications for, 82
for joint contractures, 81–86
joints requiring, 82

Catheter(s)
central venous, in head-injured patients, 6–7
Swan-Ganz, in head-injured patients, 7

Cavus, surgery for, 171, 172f

Cervical lordosis, 124, 125f

Cherney, L.R., 100

Chest tubes, in head-injured patients, 6

Cognition
definitions of, 10
evaluation of, in head-injured patients, 10–13
following brain injury, categories of, 37–38
in loss of range of motion, 81

Cognitive functioning, levels of, 11–12, 12t

Cognitive impairments
following brain injury, 35–37, 36t
serial casting and, 82

Cognitive rehabilitation, 33–54, 204
closed, 46, 46f
disability levels in, 37–39
feedback in, 48–49
functional outcome determination in, 35
handicap determination in, 37–39
meaning of, 50–51, 50t, 51t, 52f–53f
motor skill acquisition in, 44–48, 45f–47f
open, 46–47, 46f, 47f
practice in, 49
treatment management, 39–44

behavioral strategies, 39–42, 40t, 41f
learning strategies, 42–44
levels of, 39
WHO classification system in, 34, 34t

Cognitive status, in wheelchair selection and positioning evaluation, 119–120

Collagen fibers, physiologic changes in, following brain injury, 80

Community integration
components of, 201–208
conceptual issues, 201
course of treatment, 206–207
diagnostic considerations, 205–206, 205t
establishing functional treatment goals, 201–202
evaluation of outcome, 208
learning potential, 202–203
termination of treatment, 203–204
following acute rehabilitation for traumatic brain injury, 199–209. *See also* Community integration, components of.
re-entry programs in, 200, 200t

Community Integration Questionnaire (CIQ), 208

Community mobility, 205, 205t

Compensation
definition of, 57
versus movement reeducation, 56, 57–58

Composite effects, of nervous system pathology, definition of, 2

Compression boots, pneumatic, in head-injured patients, 8

Connective tissues, physiologic changes in, following brain injury, 80

Contracture(s)
adduction, of the hip, 162–163
flexion. *See* Flexion contracture.

Cough, assessment of, in swallowing dysfunction, 106–107

Curling of the toes, surgery for, 171

Defensive patients, orally, swallowing dysfunction treatment in, 109

Deformity. *See also specific types.*
fixed, 119, 122f
flexible, 119, 120f, 121f

Dentition, swallowing dysfunction and, 104

Diazepam, indications for and actions of, 5t

Dilantin, indications for and actions of, 5t

Diphosphonates, for heterotopic ossification, 93

Direct effect, of nervous system pathology, definition of, 2

Disability, definition of, 199

Discharge planning, delays in, effect on treatment, 28

Distal interphalangeal joint, limited extension of, nonfunctional surgery for, 190–191

Dolophine, indications for and actions of, 5t

Dorsal Ankle Foot Orthosis, modification of, 151, 155f, 156f

Dropout cast, 83–85, 84f
  edema and, 85
  of the leg, 163, 164f

Duncan, W., 139, 141

Dynamic splints
  advantages of, 87
  for joint contractures, 86–88
  versus serial casts, 86–87

Edema
  cast misapplication and, 86
  and dropout casts, 85

Elastic response, 87

Elbow
  heterotopic ossification at, 93
  residual deformities of
    nonfunctional surgery for, 180, 183, 184f–185f
    surgery for, 187

Elbow flexors, clonic, surgery for, 187

Electrical stimulation, intraoral, for soft palate and posterior pharyngeal wall dysfunction, 111–112, 112f

Electric mat table, in forced-use progression, 62, 63f

Environment
  effect on treatment, 29
  predictability of, in skill classification, 46–48, 46f, 47f

Equinovarus
  surgery for, 175–177, 176f
  in wheelchair seating, 134

Equinus
  surgery for, 166, 168
  in wheelchair seating, 134

Etidronate (Didronel), indications for and actions of, 5t

Exercise(s), range of motion, 24–25

Extremities
  lower. *See also* Lower extremities.
    orthotic management of, 137–160. *See also* Ankle-foot orthosis.
    in wheelchair seating, 134–135
  upper. *See also* Upper extremities.
    in wheelchair seating, 134–136

Feedback
  in cognitive rehabilitation, 48–49
  definition of, 48

Feeding program, for brain-injured patients, 113–114

Felsenthal, G., 91

Femur, positioning of, in wheelchair seating, 132–133

Fentanyl (Sublimaze), indications for and actions of, 5t

Fingers
  Boutonniere deformities of, nonfunctional surgery for, 192, 193f
  intrinsic plus deformities of, nonfunctional surgery for, 192
  limited extension of, 189, 191f
  residual deformities of
    nonfunctional surgery for, 183–184, 186f
    surgery for, 189–192, 191f, 193f, 194f

First ray mobilization, 143, 146f, 147f

Flexion contracture
  of the elbow, nonfunctional surgery for, 180, 183, 184f–185f
  of the fingers, nonfunctional surgery for, 183–184
  of the hip, nonfunctional surgery for, 162–163, 162f
  of the knee, nonfunctional surgery for, 163, 164f
  of the proximal interphalangeal joint, nonfunctional surgery for, 191
  of the wrist, nonfunctional surgery for, 183–184

Flexion deformity, of the wrist, nonfunctional surgery for, 184–185

Fluoroscopy, swallowing, 107

Foam wedges, 21, 23f

Foot
  bones of, 139, 140f
  mobilization of, 142–146, 144f–147f. *See also* Mobilization, ankle and foot.
  neurobiologic assessment of, 141
  normal, structural alignment and function in, 139–141, 140f
  planovalgus, surgery for, 169–170, 170f
  plantar surfaces of, in postural grounding, 138
  problems of, case studies, 147–160, 149f–159f
  residual deformities of, surgery for, 175–176, 177f
  tonic reflexes of, 139, 141

Foot boards, 21, 21f, 22, 23f

Foot splints, polypropylene, 21, 22f

Forced-use intervention
  clinical hypotheses in, 71–75, 73f
  preparation for, 67–71, 69f
  in restoration of motor control, 60–75, 63f–69f, 73f

Forefoot, residual deformities of, surgery for, 168–171, 170f

Forefoot-heel-ankle varus, surgery for, 171, 173f

Forefoot varus, surgery for, 168–169
Fralish, K., 204
Fryer, J., 204
Functional activities approach in cognitive
    rehabiitation, 204

Glasgow Coma Scale, 10–11, 11t
    Ranchos Los Amigos Levels of Cognitive
        Functioning (LOC) Scale and, relationship
        between, 13
Goal formulation, 19–20, 19t
Gordon, J., 58, 59f, 65

Haloperidol (Haldol), indications for and actions of,
    5t
Halo strap, 132
Halper, A.S., 100
Hamstrings, hypertonic, surgery for, 166, 167f
Hand(s), palmar surfaces of, in postural grounding,
    138
Handicap, definition of, 199–200
Hand opening, voluntary, with limited extension,
    188f
Head alignment
    deficits in, swallowing dysfunction treatment
        and, 108–109
    maintenance of, in evaluation of swallowing
        structures, 101–102
    in wheelchair seating, 130–132
Head injury(ies)
    acute care hospital management of, 1–31
        airway management, 3, 5
        arterial lines in, 7
        central venous catheters in, 6–7
        chest tubes in, 6
        cognitive evaluation, 10–13
        discharge planning, 26
        external devices used in, 21–24, 21f–24f
        focus of, 1–2
        goal formulation, 19–20, 19t
        incidence of, 1
        intermittent pneumatic calf-compression
            boots in, 8
        intracranial pressure monitors in, 7–8
        medical record review, 2–3, 4f
        motor control evaluation, 13–18
        motor output evaluation, 16
        movement facilitation, 25, 25f–27f
        muscle tone evaluation, 15–16
        musculoskeletal evaluation, 13–15, 15t
        nutritional, 6
        observation of movement, 9
        obstacles associated with, 26–28

        patient evaluation, 2–18
        patient observation, 3, 5–8
        patient positioning in, 9, 21, 21f–24f, 24
        peripheral intravenous lines in, 6
        pulmonary artery lines in, 7
        pulmonary care, 20–21
        pulmonary system evaluation, 9–10
        range of motion/relaxation techniques, 24–25
        reflexive motor behavior evaluation, 16–17
        survival following, 1
        voluntary motor behavior evaluation, 17–18,
            18f
    hospitalization for, 1
    incidence of, 1
    mortality due to, 1
Head supports, wheelchair, 130–131
Heel, residual deformities of, surgery for, 168, 169f
Heel varus, surgery for, 168, 169f
Heterotopic ossification
    definition of, 92
    diphosphonates in, 93
    following brain injury, 92–96
    joint manipulation for, 93
    range-of-motion exercises for, 93–96
    sites for, 93–94
Hierarchical task approach in cognitive
    rehabilitation, 204
Hip
    adduction contracture of, surgery for, 162–163
    flexion contracture of, surgery for, 162, 162f
    heterotopic ossification at, 93–94
    residual deformities of
        nonfunctional surgery for, 162–163, 162f
        surgery for, 164–165, 165f
Hip adductors, hypertonic, surgery for, 164–165
Hip alignment, in wheelchair seating, 132–133
Hip extensors, hypertonic, surgery for, 164, 165f

Impairment
    definition of, 199
    Disability, Handicap, (IDH) model, 199
Indirect effect, of nervous system pathology,
    definition of, 2
Instrumental skills approach in cognitive
    rehabilitation, 204
Intensive care unit (ICU), neurologic
    acute care management in, 1–31. *See also* Head in-
        jury(ies), acute care hospital management of
    medications used in, 5t
Internal rotation of the shoulder, nonfunctional
    surgery for, 180, 181f
Interphalangeal joint
    distal, limited extension of, 190–191
    proximal

flexion contracture of, 191
   surgery for, 172–173, 174f
Intracranial pressure (ICP) monitors, in head-injured patients, 7–8
Intraoral sensory examination, swallowing dysfunction and, 103–104
Intrinsic plus deformities
   nonfunctional surgery for, 192
   surgery for, 173–174, 175f
Intubation, tracheal, in head-injured patients, 5
Investment principles, in restoration of motor control, 58–60, 59f
Ischial tuberosities, 126, 126f
   of the pelvis, in postural grounding, 138

Jennett, B., 10, 11t
Johnston, M.V., 208
Joint contracture(s)
   definition of, 80
   dynamic splints for, 86–88
   following brain injury, 79–81
   orthotic management of, 88–89
   serial casting for, 81–86
   surgery for, 91–92
Joint manipulation, for heterotopic ossification, 93
Jordan, P., 139

Kinetic chain, definition of, 138
Knee
   flexion contracture of, surgery for, 163, 164f
   heterotopic ossification at, 93
   positioning of, in wheelchair seating, 134
   residual deformities of
      nonfunctional surgery for, 163, 164f
      surgery for, 165–166, 167f
Knee-ankle-foot orthoses (KAFO), 88
Kyphosis, thoracic, 124, 125f

Larynx, control of
   deficits in, 112–113
   swallowing dysfunction and, 105–106
Lazarus, C.L., 100
Leahy, P., 37
Learned nonuse syndrome, 56
Learning
   versus performance, 43
   phases of, 44
Learning ability, definition of, 43
Learning potential, in rehabilitation process, 202–203
Learning treatment strategies, 42–44
Leg, dropout cast of, 163, 164f

LeVere, T.E., 57
Lewis, F., 208
Lidocaine (Xylocaine)
   indications for and actions of, 5t
   for spasticity, 89–91
Ligament(s), physiologic changes in, following brain injury, 80
Limbs, mobility of, for forced-use progression therapy, 67–70, 69f
Lioresal, indications for and actions of, 5t
Logemann, J.A., 100
Lorazepam, indications for and actions of, 5t
Lordosis
   cervical, 124, 125f
   lumbar, 124, 125f
Lower extremities. *See also* Ankle; Foot; Hip; Knee; Toes.
   equinovarus deformity of, 175–177, 176f
   orthotic management of, 137–160. *See also* Ankle-foot orthosis.
   residual deformities of
      functional surgery for, 163–177
      nonfunctional surgery for, 161–163, 162f
      reconstructive surgery for, 161–177. *See also* *specific site, e.g.,* Hip.
Lumbar lordosis, 124, 125f

Malex, J.F., 208
Mannitol, indications for and actions of, 5t
Medical acuity, effect on treatment, 27
Medical record, review of, in head-injured patients, 2–3, 4f
Medical status, in wheelchair selection and positioning evaluation, 119
Memory loss, handicaps related to, 34t
Merrit, D., 151
Merrit, P.T., 151
Methadone, indications for and actions of, 5t
Metocurine iodine, indications for and actions of, 5t
Metubine, indications for and actions of, 5t
Midtarsal joint mobilization, 143, 146f
Mobility, of the limbs, for forced-use progression therapy, 67–70, 69f
Mobilization, ankle and foot, 142–146, 144f–147f
   first ray, 143, 146f, 147f
   midtarsal, 143, 146f
   subtalar, 143, 145f
   tibio-talar, 142–143, 144f
Motor behavior
   automatic, 18, 18f
   conscious, 17
   movements in, 45–46, 45f
   reflexive
      definition of, 16

Motor behavior *(Continued)*
  evaluation of, 16–17
  voluntary
    definition of, 17
    evaluation of, 17–18, 18f
Motor control
  evaluation of, in head-injured patients, 13–18
  restoration of, 55–78
    clinical hypotheses in, 71–75, 73f
    forced-use paradigm/progression in, 60–75,
      63f–69f, 73f
    investment principles in, 58–60, 59f
    preparation for, 67–71, 69f
    task-specific training in, 75–76
Motor learning, definition of, 43
Motor output, evaluation of, in head-injured
  patients, 16
Motor performance, definition of, 43
Motor point block, for spasticity, 89–91
Motor skills
  acquisition of, 44–48, 45f–47f
  definition of, 44
Movement(s)
  abnormal, versus spasticity, 81
  continence, 46
  discrete, 45, 45f
  facilitation of, devices used in, 25, 25f–27f
  in head-injured patients, observation of, 9
  linkage of, in restoration of motor control, 63,
    66f–68f
  serial, 45
Movement control, loss of, handicaps related to, 34t
Movement dysfunction
  definition of, 121
  fixed, 119, 122f
  in wheelchair selection and positioning
    evaluation, 120–123
Movement reeducation, versus compensation, 56,
  57–58
Movement strategies, transitional, orthoses for, 137
Muscle fibers, physiologic changes in, following
  brain injury, 80
Muscle tone, evaluation of, in head-injured patients,
  15–16
Musculoskeletal system
  in head-injured patients, evaluation of, 13–15,
    15t
  impairments of, in head-injured patients, 13–15,
    15t

Neck alignment
  maintenance of, in evaluation of swallowing
    structures, 101–102
  in wheelchair seating, 130–132

Nembutal, indications for and actions of, 5t
Nerve blocks
  in residual lower extremity deformity evaluation,
    161
  for spasticity, 89–91
Neurological Intensive Care Unit Vital Sign Flow
  Sheet, 3, 4f
Norton, B.J., 81
Nutritional support, in head-injured patients, 6

Orally defensive patients, swallowing dysfunction
  treatment in, 109
Oral-phase control, swallowing dysfunction
  treatment and, 110
Oral reflexes, heightened, swallowing dysfunction
  treatment and, 109
Orofacial structures, assessment of
  dentition, 104
  intraoral responses and sensation, 103–104
  response to cutaneous stimulation, 102–103
  soft palate and posterior pharyngeal wall, 105
  strength and mobility of the perioral structures,
    103
  swallowing dysfunction and, 102–105
  tongue control, 104–105
Orthoses
  ankle-foot. *See* Ankle-foot orthosis.
  for joint contractures, 88–89
  lower extremity, 137–160. *See also* Ankle-foot
    orthosis.
  purpose of, 137
  types of, 88–89
  Utley Foot Orthosis (UFO), 142, 149, 149f–151f
Ossification, heterotopic, following brain injury,
  92–96. *See also* Heterotopic ossification,
  following brain injury.
Outrigger devices, for casts, 85
Oxygen, partial pressure of, normal, 20
Oxygen saturation, normal, levels of, 20

Pancuronium bromide, indications for and actions
  of, 5t
Paresis, handicaps related to, 34t
Patient observation, 3, 5–8
Patient positioning, in head-injured patients, 9, 21,
  21f–24f, 24
Pavulon, indications for and actions of, 5t
Pelvis, ischial tuberosities of, in postural grounding,
  138
Pentobarbital, indications for and actions of, 5t
Pentothal, indications for and actions of, 5t
Perceptual acuity, in wheelchair selection and
  positioning evaluation, 120

Perceptual deficits, handicaps related to, 34t
Performance, versus learning, 43
Peripheral intravenous lines, in head-injured
        patients, 6
Pharyngeal wall
    inadequate function of, swallowing dysfunction
        treatment and, 110–112, 112f
    posterior, assessment of, 105
Phenobarbital, indications for and actions of, 5t
Phenol
    effects on nerves, 91
    for spasticity, 89–91
        indications for, 90
        open injection, 91
        percutaneous injection, 91
        purpose of, 90
        site for, 91
Phenytoin, indications for and actions of, 5t
Physical condition, following brain injury,
        categories of, 38
Planovalgus foot, surgery for, 169–170, 170f
Plastic response, 87
Pole(s), bedside, uses of, 25, 26f
Postural control factors, 137
Postural grounding, 138–139
    definition of, 138
Practice
    blocked, 49
    in cognitive rehabilitation, 49
    random, 49
Procaine, in residual lower extremity deformity
        evaluation, 161
Progression
    definition of, 62
    forced-use, 60–75, 63f–69f, 73f
Propranolol (Inderal), indications for and actions
        of, 5t
Proximal interphalangeal joint
    flexion contracture of, nonfunctional surgery for,
        191
    flexion of, surgery for, 172–173, 174f
Pulmonary artery lines, in head-injured patients, 7
Pulmonary system
    evaluation of, in head-injured patients, 9–10
    management of, in head-injured patients, 20–21

Quadriceps, hypertonic, surgery for, 165–166

Ranchos Los Amigos Levels of Cognitive
        Functioning (LOC) Scale, 11–12, 12t, 37
    Glasgow Coma Scale and, relationship between,
        13
Range of motion activities, 68–70, 69f

Range of motion exercises, 24–25
    for heterotopic ossification, 93–96
Range of motion (ROM)
    assessment of, 80
        of ankle and foot, 1451
    decreased
        cognitive effect on, 81
        in head-injured patients, 14–15, 15t
        management of, 79–97
    functional, in wheelchair selection and
        positioning evaluation, 119
Reconstructive surgery
    for residual lower extremity deformities,
        161–177. *See also specific site, e.g.*, Hip.
    for residual upper extremity deformities,
        179–197. *See also specific site, e.g.,* Wrist.
Rehabilitation
    cognitive, 33–54. *See also* Cognitive
        rehabilitation.
    lack of understanding of the benefits of, effect on
        treatment, 27–28
Rehabilitation outcome, successful, 35
Resting cast, 82
Rooting response, 102

Sahgal, V., 13
Sahrmann, S.A., 81
Schenkman, M., 2
Schmidt, N., 151
Scoliosis, flexible, 119, 120f, 121f
Sensory loss, handicaps related to, 34t
Shoulder
    heterotopic ossification at, 93
    internal rotation of, nonfunctional surgery for,
        180, 181f
    residual deformities of, nonfunctional surgery
        for, 180, 181f
    subluxation of, nonfunctional surgery for, 180,
        182f
Skills
    acquisition of
        definition of, 44
        in forced-use progression, 65
    classification of, 46–48, 46f, 47f
    definition of, 43
Skin breakdown, cast misapplication and, 86
Soft palate
    assessment of, in swallowing dysfunction,
        105
    inadequate function of, in swallowing
        dysfunction treatment, 110–112, 112f
Spasticity
    abnormal movement and, relationship between,
        81

Spasticity *(Continued)*
  botulinim toxin for, 92
  components of, 80
  definition of, 80
  evaluation of, 80
  motor point blocks for, 89–91
  nerve blocks for, 89–91
  reduction in
    bupivacaine for, 89–90
    lidocaine for, 89–90
    phenol for, 89–91
  in wheelchair seating, 135
Spinal curves, 124–125, 125f–127f
Splints
  air, 21
  dynamic
    advantage of, 87
    for joint contractures, 86–88
    versus serial casts, 86–87
  foot, polypropylene, 21, 22f
Spontaneous recovery, 56
Spreader bars, for casts, 85
Stool stepping, in forced-use progression, 62–63,
      63f–65f
Strip casts, with bilateral toe-spreaders, 156
Subluxation of the shoulder, nonfunctional surgery
      for, 180, 182f
Subtalar joint mobilization, 143, 145f
Surgery
  functional
    indications for, 163, 185–186
    for residual lower extremity deformities,
      163–177
    for residual upper extremity deformities,
      185–196
  nonfunctional
    reasons for, 161
    for residual lower extremity deformities,
      161–163, 162f
    for residual upper extremity deformities,
      179–185, 181f, 182f, 184f, 185f
Swallowing dysfunction, 99–115
  feeding program for, 113–114
  incidence of, 100
  patient evaluation, 100–107
    assessment of the head, neck, and trunk
      control, 101–102
    of cough, 106–107
    laryngeal control, 105–106
    medical record review, 101
    orofacial examination, 102–105. *See also*
      Orofacial structures, assessment of.
    physical examination, 101
    swallowing fluoroscopy in, 107
  treatment for, 108–113

for head and trunk control deficits, 108–109
for inadequate function of the soft palate and
    posterior pharyngeal wall, 110–112, 112f
for laryngeal control deficits, 112–113
in patients with oral defensiveness or
    heightened oral reflexes, 109
promoting improved control of oral-phase
    function, 110
Swallowing fluoroscopy, 107
Swan-Ganz catheters, in head-injured patients, 7
Szekeres, S.F., 207

Task-specific training, in restoration of motor
    control, 75–76
Taub, E., 56
Teasdale, G., 10, 11t
Teeth, examination of, swallowing dysfunction and,
    104
Thiopental, indications for and actions of, 5t
Thoracic kyphosis, 124, 125f
Thumb, residual deformities of, nonfunctional
    surgery for, 192–196, 194f–196f
Thumb in palm deformities, nonfunctional surgery
    for, 193–196, 194f–196f
Tibio-talar mobilization, 142–143, 144f
Tilt table, 22–23, 24f
Toe(s)
  curling of, surgery for, 171
  residual deformities of, surgery for, 171–174,
    174f, 175–176, 175f, 177f
Toe-spreader, 151, 154f
  strip casts with, 156
Tongue, control of, swallowing dysfunction and,
    104–105
Tonic reflexes, of the foot, 139, 141
Training, in forced-use progression, 65
Treatment plan, 19t, 20–25
Trunk, lower, stretching of, 69f
Trunk alignment
  deficits in, swallowing dysfunction treatment
    and, 108–109
  maintenance of, in evaluation of swallowing
    structures, 101–102
  in wheelchair seating, 128f, 129–130, 130f, 131f
  in wheelchair selection and positioning
    evaluation, 122f–128f, 124–127

Upper extremities. *See also* Elbow; Fingers;
    Hands; Shoulder; Thumb, Wrist.
  residual deformities of
    functional surgery for, 185–196
    nonfunctional surgery for, 179–185, 181f,
      182f, 184f, 185f

reconstructive surgery for, 179–197. *See also specific sites.*
Utley Foot Orthosis (UFO), 142, 148, 149f–151f

Valium, indications for and actions of, 5t
Vecuronium bromide (Norcuron), indications for and actions of, 5t
Visual acuity, in wheelchair selection and positioning evaluation, 120

Weight shift, process of, 69f
Wheelchair(s), selection of, 123–124
Wheelchair seating
  proper positioning for, 117–136
    assessment of, 119–123, 120f–122f
    hip joint alignment, 132–133
    lower extremity alignment, 134–135
    optimization of, 117–119
    spasticity and, 135

trunk alignment, 122f–128f, 124–127
upper extremity alignment, 134–136
setting up the system, 127–136
  head and neck alignment, 130–132
  trunk alignment, 128f, 129–130, 130f, 131f
WHO. *See* World Health Organization *and* Wrist-hand orthosis.
Willer, B., 208
Winstein, C.J., 100
World Health Organization (WHO) classification for brain injury, 34, 34t
  definitions of, 199–200
Wrist
  limited extension of, surgery for, 187, 188f–189f
  limited flexion of, surgery for, 187, 189, 190f
  residual deformities of
    nonfunctional surgery for, 183–185, 186f
    surgery for, 187–189, 188f–190f
Wrist-hand orthosis (WHO), 89

Yarkony, G., 13